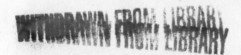

# *The Enchanted Ring*

# The Enchanted Ring
## The Untold Story of Penicillin

John C. Sheehan

The MIT Press
Cambridge, Massachusetts
London, England

Second printing, 1982
© 1982 by
John C. Sheehan

This book was set in Baskerville by Achorn Graphic Services, Inc., and printed and bound by The Murray Printing Co. in the United States of America.

Library of Congress Cataloging in Publication Data

Sheehan, John C.
    The enchanted ring.

    Bibliography: p.
    Includes index.
    1. Penicillin—History.  I. Title.
RM666.P35S47      615'.32923      82-2093
ISBN  0-262-19204-7                    AACR2

# Contents

# *Foreword*

A number of books and many popular articles have been written about the history of penicillin and those who had a part in it. Most of them begin with Fleming's discovery and terminate with the introduction of penicillin into clinical medicine by Florey and his colleagues more than ten years later. More often than not, the authors have no personal knowledge of what had happened, and the reliance of some of them on hearsay has led to fantasies that bear little resemblance to the facts. The task of the serious historian here has not been an easy one, for irreconcilable differences of opinion between the main characters became apparent at an early stage. Thus it has never been possible to present the history of penicillin in a way that would have been pleasing to all those concerned.

Professor Sheehan's book is one man's story of the penicillin molecule, with its enchanted beta-lactam ring, and differs in several respects from its predecessors. It presents the vital but sometimes neglected contributions of Americans to the production of penicillin in quantity during World War II and it reveals the little advertised role of chemistry in the developments that occurred during this time and the following two decades. The author is an organic chemist of distinction, known for his outstanding achievements in the penicillin field. After the war, when the efforts of more than a thousand chemists in thirty-nine major laboratories in Britain and the United States had failed to produce penicillin by an acceptable chemical synthesis, he alone took up the challenge of what seemed then to be a daunting and perhaps insoluble problem. By systematic research extending over more than a decade at the Massachusetts Institute of Technology, he was able to show that the problem had a rational solution. I still remember the day when Sir Robert Robinson telephoned to tell me, with noticeable excitement, that John Sheehan was in Oxford and that he had described a total synthesis of penicillin.

Years later, when Sir Robert was eighty-six years old, almost totally blind, and nearing the end of his life, he asked me to collaborate with him in writing a book on the chemistry of penicillin. "We shall be able," he said, with something like a chuckle, "to put the Americans in their place." For reasons that were not entirely concerned with Anglo-American chemical relationships, I viewed this proposal with some alarm and was relieved when it came to nothing. But it had long been evident that claims to priority for some of the findings that first threw light on the nature of penicillin could become subjects of misunderstanding. They had been recorded in secret reports, exchanged between London and Washington, that suffered long delays in transit. This gave time enough for the same discoveries to be made independently on each side of the Atlantic.

It was about this time that John Sheehan told me that he hoped to write the penicillin story, "especially from the U.S. point of view and the more recent developments." Having recently written a memoir on those parts of the story that centered around Lord Florey, I replied that it would be nice if he could fill in some of the other parts of the picture. In *The Enchanted Ring* this has been done and an American viewpoint vividly portrayed. We can read about deliberations in the Nobel Committee of 1945 that eventually divided a prize between Fleming, Florey, and Chain, and about the problems of the wartime Committee on Medical Research of the Office of Scientific Research and Development in Washington when it was assigned the role of coordinating research on penicillin production and synthesis in the United States and maintaining a liaison with The Medical Research Council in London. We learn of the credit due to those in the Northern Regional Research Laboratory of the U.S. Department of Agriculture at Peoria and to the firms of Merck, Squibb, Pfizer, and others, by whose efforts the formidable problem of producing penicillin G in quantity was overcome. We are told of the immense body of research on the chemical aspects of penicillin, little known to the public, that laid foundations for some of the remarkable advances in the chemotherapy of bacterial infections that have been made since penicillin first became available to the physician. And we are given a personal view of the story of the penicillin nucleus, 6-aminopenicillanic acid, which was obtained in Sheehan's laboratory by chemical synthesis in 1956–1957 and then in the Beecham Laboratories by fermentation, and which became a key substance in the production of new penicillins of clinical value.

Superimposed on the microbiological and chemical achievements described in this book were human and legal problems. John Sheehan makes it clear that the friction generated by early events in the history of penicillin in Britain was paralleled in the United States by dissatisfaction about the relative status and rewards of those in academic, federal, and commercial organizations and was followed by a lengthy international dispute about patents. Perhaps this was an almost inevitable consequence of the interaction of human frailty with a highly complex situation in which there were great prizes, both academic and financial. Nevertheless, the production and development of penicillin G and of new penicillins for use in human medicine has had a success that would have seemed unbelievable when Florey carried out his first therapeutic experiments.

John Sheehan has made extensive use of contemporary documents. He will scarcely expect that all those who read his book will purr with approval of the contents of every page, for on some of his topics there may never be a final word. But controversy can add relish to a story told at first hand and it does so here. The book is eminently readable and throws light on exciting and hitherto unfamiliar facets of the penicillin saga.

Sir Edward Abraham

# *Preface*

I have several reasons for telling the story of penicillin. Not the least of them is that through forty years of penicillin research, I came to know some of the greatest scientists of our time. Abraham, Bachmann, Barton, Bose, Chain, Clarke, Fleming, Florey, Folkers, Foster, Hodgkin, Keefer, Robinson, Tishler, du Vigneaud, Wintersteiner, Woodward, and many others. Although the story I am about to tell is about the chemical synthesis of penicillin from simple raw materials, it is more generally about the growth of industrial and academic science during the years of World War II and immediately after. These were years during which science came to occupy a central position in American life and polity. The penicillin project was one of the signal events of that history.

Moreover, the complete story of penicillin has not yet been told. There is far more to the penicillin story than Fleming's master stroke in 1928. There is more to the story than the important work done by Sir Howard Florey, Dr. Ernst B. Chain, Dr. E. P. Abraham, and Dr. N. G. Heatley during the 1930s and 1940s. The story that has been told, to date, is predominantly the story of the British contribution to penicillin. There is an important American side to that same story.

Government, university, and commercial interests cooperated in producing the naturally fermented penicillins and worked together toward the possible synthesis. All participants in this project waived their rights to patents until, at the end of the war, government agencies would oversee the equitable distribution of patent rights. How this industrial arrangement was created is a story as complex as that of the penicillin synthesis itself. Until now that story has remained locked in the private files of the Office of Scientific Research and Development (OSRD) and its Committee on Medical Research (CMR). Other records remained in the archives of the National Academy of Sciences and its Committee on Chemotherapeutic and Other Agents. These two groups in particular had prime responsibility for developing naturally fermented penicillins and for governing the research toward the synthesis of a penicillin.

The documents are marked SECRET and have remained so since the close of World War II. They reveal a story of cooperation between government and private industry, aided by the academic scientific community, that could not be repeated today. Laws have changed, customs are different, and the United States is no longer the small country it was before World War II. The club that organized and directed the penicillin program no longer exists. This book, therefore, tells the story of one of the final chapters in the history of that club.

All was not sweetness and light. The agreement to cooperate was difficult to forge and, once the agreement was sketched, it was difficult to enforce. Throughout the complex and trying period of the penicillin project, dissent threatened to upset major parts of the program. Patent claims were critical issues even in the earliest years of the penicillin program. They have remained so. Great sums of money have changed hands in the buying and selling of penicillin, in the open market and in the black market. The story of the wonder drug, consequently, also involves the story of proprietary rights and royalties, dollars and the promise of dollars. In my own case, after having successfully synthesized penicillin in 1957, the patent situation was not cleared up until April 1980, after twenty-three years of contention.

I am telling the story of penicillin, too, because I have witnessed most of the major developments over the past forty years and have participated in many of them.

One secret intelligence report dispatched from the United States to Great Britain during World War II commented, "Penicillin is surging upwards and is going to have a tremendous vogue here. I am hearing about it from many people" (J. H. Burn, *Newsletter* No. 28, May 31, 1943). In particular, the interest of military medical men in treating battle injuries and combating the rampant venereal disease that accompanies any army promoted interest in the wonder drug. With "lightning rapidity," according to the popular press at the time, penicillin "shot into the front ranks of therapeutic agents," displacing the sulfa drugs from their "exalted position" (*New Republic* 109(1943):20–21).

Penicillin was endowed with almost magical powers. And, as is the case with any incantation, the spell must be pronounced properly. On October 25, 1943, "a group of scientists voting on the pronunciation of the term" decided by a margin of 70 to 30 percent that penicillin should be pronounced peniCILLin and not penICillin (*Drug Trade News* 18(1943):28). As Moses could look down from Mount Pisgah, so Americans congratulated themselves on their discovery of "a new promised land in medicine" (*New York Times,* September 10, 1943) in which all pathological germs would be destroyed by the new "life-saving weapon."

Penicillin was a technical triumph that captured the imagination of a public far beyond the boundaries of the laboratory and the hospital. The magic of the substance endowed the people associated with it with glamor. Scientists studying penicillin became popular heroes; doctors who administered it became holy men; and, at least during the war years when penicillin was in desperately short supply, the man who controlled its distribution became a god.

Here is the story of that drug—the efforts to develop Fleming's discovery and the scientific program to develop penicillin into an effective and commercially successful chemotherapeutic agent.

# Acknowledgments

Several people have generously contributed their time and energy to this book. The following have allowed me to tape-record their recollections of penicillin research:

Sir Edward Abraham, Sir William Dunn Laboratory of Pathology, Oxford University

Jack Baldwin, Dyson Perrins Laboratory, Oxford University

Sir Derek Barton, Central Laboratory for Natural Science, Gif sur Yvette, formerly of Imperial College, London

Sir Ernst Chain, Imperial College, London

Arnold L. Demain, Massachusetts Institute of Technology

Karl Folkers, University of Texas, formerly of Merck Sharp & Dohme

Dame Dorothy Hodgkin, Oxford University

Amel R. Menotti, Bristol Laboratories

Robert Morin, Bristol Laboratories, formerly of Eli Lilly

Jack Strominger, Harvard University

Max Tishler, Wesleyan University, formerly of Merck Sharp & Dohme

Hamao Umezawa, Institute for Microbial Chemistry, Tokyo

I have also profited immensely from frequent conversations with

Ajay K. Bose, Stevens Institute of Technology

Sir Ewart Jones, Oxford University, president of the Royal Institute of Chemistry

Dagmar Ponzi, Massachusetts Institute of Technology

The Lord Todd, Cambridge University, president of The Royal Society

Robert Burns Woodward, Harvard University

Robert N. Ross, director of the Graduate Program in Science Communication, Boston University, assisted in the preparation of the manuscript.

My brother, Joseph G. Sheehan of the University of California, Los Angeles, provided valuable counsel at formative stages of the book.

# 1 The Lonely Search

I have often been asked why I undertook to synthesize penicillin after the most extensive and intensive effort in the history of organic chemistry, indeed of all medical science, had failed. Only the Manhattan Project leading to the development of the atomic bomb equaled the efforts of the Office of Scientific Research and Development during World War II to produce a synthetic penicillin. When the penicillin project failed to accomplish this goal, most research directors in the pharmaceutical industry and academic chemists in the universities were led to the conclusion that the synthesis of penicillin was an impossible problem.

For several years a synthetic penicillin had seemed just within reach. In the early days of the research program, chemists optimistically thought that because penicillin was a small molecule, synthesizing the compound would pose no special problems. However, although chemists working in the United States and Great Britain did in time describe the characteristic chemistry of penicillin and, after much disagreement and confusion, even worked out the structure of the penicillin molecule, they failed in their primary goal: to design a rational process for synthesizing penicillin. The penicillin molecule proved to be trickier than that generation of chemists had suspected. After many years of intensive research, most investigators involved in the study of penicillin felt that even if a successful synthesis were finally designed, that feat would probably never amount to more than a clever scientific stunt. In any event, according to most authorities on penicillin in the late 1940s and early 1950s, the naturally fermented penicillins would continue to dominate the field. They were plentiful and, as far as anyone knew at the time, they probably could not be surpassed.

Mine was a lonely search for the right combination of materials and methods by which to make a penicillin in the laboratory. After their own tentative efforts to continue penicillin research were frustrated, most other synthetic chemists in the field abandoned penicillin research to me. How I laid the groundwork for the synthesis of penicillin, how I recast the problem, the new tools I devised for the job are the subjects of my book.

While this is the story of penicillin, it is also a personal story of frustration and discovery. Accounts of scientific discoveries often oversimplify the bewildering complexities of research. In movie versions of science, for instance, one sees the moment at which the scientist finds the long-sought microbe under the microscope or finally discovers the hoped-for product in the test tube. In all discovery there is a moment of what psychologists call the Aha! experience. That triumph occurs in the privacy of the creative mind. Artists and scientists share that particular joy. However, there are the long periods during which the work must go on before that moment of high enthusiasm. And after the discovery, other complexities intrude themselves. If the discovery is an important one, the public soon becomes aware of it. The private triumph becomes a personal and social responsibility at that point. In my case, the struggles after I had found synthetic penicillin in my test tube were at least as arduous as the labors that preceded that exciting moment. The scientific triumph led to the development of a whole family of life-saving antibiotics. Just as important for the scientist, the successful synthesis of penicillin reaffirmed the triumph of reason in a world of disorder.

For thirty years after the discovery of a natural penicillin by Sir Alexander Fleming, the source and the nature of the penicillins changed only slightly. From the time Fleming published his discovery in 1929 through the 1930s very little new information was developed about penicillin. Today we are familiar with the wonders of antibiotics, but fifty years ago the unprecedented benefits of enlisting the penicillin molecule in the battle to destroy disease-producing organisms were only dimly perceived. Even medical experts, who might have known better, considered penicillin a minor laboratory curiosity. Despite early efforts, ten years after Fleming's discovery of penicillin in 1928, the chemical structure of penicillin had yet to be established; the substance was not available in appreciable amounts for medical therapy or for scientific research; and few people thought that antibiotics had much of a future.

World War II changed all that. The military emergency raised the medical problems of treating battlefield injuries and disease from the level of academic research to national crisis. The sulfa drugs, themselves only recently developed, were one important means of treating disease chemically; but they were limited. The sulfa drugs had a very narrow spectrum of activity; many diseases could not be treated successfully with them. Some bacteria were capable of developing resistance to sulfa drugs with alarming rapidity. Finally, the sulfa drugs could interfere with the body's own natural defense against infection. As one response to the pressing needs, the United States government undertook a large-scale effort to produce penicillin in therapeutically useful quantities. Exploratory research conducted in Great Britain by Sir Howard Florey, Dr. Ernst B. Chain, Dr. N. G. Heatley, and Dr. E. P. Abraham, all working at Oxford University, had revealed the exciting potential of penicillin. Although the Oxford team had produced only small amounts of concentrated but still impure penicillin in their laboratory, they had successfully demonstrated the value of penicillin in treating a variety of otherwise intractable diseases and had thereby extended the pioneering work done by Fleming.

As part of the wartime drive instigated by Florey and others toward improved biological production of naturally fermented penicillin, the U.S. government initiated a massive effort organized by the Office of Scientific Research and Development (OSRD), Committee on Medical Research (CMR) to determine the chemical structure of the penicillin molecule and to try to synthesize the drug by purely chemical means. The government-organized effort to produce penicillin went in two directions: one toward the maximum production of naturally fermented penicillin; the other toward the chemical synthesis of penicillins. The two projects were closely related, of course, for the raw materials of the chemical work were made possible only by the successes of the biological work.

At the height of the effort during World War II, more than thirty-nine major laboratories were involved in the efforts to synthesize penicillin. At least one thousand chemists were involved in the project. Failure was mounted upon failure, despite this massive investment by the U.S. government, private commercial interests, and academic institutions. The total chemical synthesis of penicillin came to be known—and with some justification—as the impossible problem.

The general impression current among people familiar with the history of penicillin is that British scientists deserve the full measure of credit for initial insights into the virtues of the *Penicillium* mold as well as most of the credit for describing the fundamental chemical properties of the substance penicillin. According to this popular, albeit mistaken, view of the history of penicillin, Americans were parvenues who came into penicillin research only after the German bombing of Britain made British research in penicillin difficult and industrial production practically impossible.

This view of history assigns American scientists a relatively minor role in the development of penicillin. The belief was current as early as the beginnings of the penicillin development (*British Medical Journal,* August 5, 1942, p. 186; Levaditi, 1945). The British were given credit for the scientific insight; the Americans were thanked for their industrial ingenuity.

One of the American pioneers in penicillin research tried to correct this misconception at the source. He agreed that the work of the British researchers should be recognized, but, he wrote, "I would not be satisfied with my attempt to review the historical development of penicillin if I failed to correct the impression, which prevails to some degree, that scientists in this country were not intensively interested in penicillin before our government agencies, stimulated by Florey's visit [June 1941], became actively engaged in sponsoring its development" (Herrell, p. 8).

At least three major scientific projects involving penicillin were already in progress before representatives of the Oxford group enlisted the aid of the Americans in the summer of 1941. In 1930, Roger D. Reid, working at the Pennsylvania State College, compared cultures of twenty-three molds with subcultures of Fleming's original *Penicillium notatum* "to find others than the one isolated by Fleming which would produce a similar inhibitory substance" ("Some properties of a bacterial-inhibitory substance produced by a mold," *Journal of Bacteriology* 29(1935):215–221). None but Fleming's mold did. In 1940 and 1941, workers at Beth Israel Hospital and Columbia Medical College in New York and the Mayo Clinic in Rochester, Minnesota, had begun serious studies of the chemistry of penicillin and its chemotherapeutic action.

The general impression is mistaken in another respect as well. One would be led to believe that a cadre of American technicians, mobilized by the United States government during the hectic preparations for war and motivated by the industrial instinct for profit, had nothing more sophisticated to do than scale up the small laboratory procedures developed by the British to full-blown industrial production.

This impression is far from what actually happened in those difficult years of the early 1940s.

Even when the time came for the industrial production of penicillin, countless questions remained unanswered. What was the structure of the penicillin molecule? What were the most effective ways of isolating penicillin from the fermentation broth in which it was produced? What were the most appropriate methods for growing the mold? And, ultimately, could the drug be synthesized?

Of course commercial interests influenced the development of penicillin. Those same commercial interests, however, required the most sophisticated fundamental research into the microbiology of the *Penicillium* mold and the chemistry of its most important product.

It was known that the penicillins were relatively small molecules, with molecular weights of about 350. That was encouraging, for the relatively low molecular weight put penicillin well within the range of molecules that had already been synthesized by industrial processes. Unfortunately, we soon realized that the size of the molecule was the least of our problems in working with penicillin. From the point of view of the organic chemist, penicillin was a molecule that was far ahead of its time. The fact that a thousand of the best chemists in the United States and Great Britain could not come up with a definitive synthesis of penicillin did not reflect upon their unquestioned abilities. Rather it indicated to me that the appropriate techniques and reactions for putting together the penicillin molecule simply had not yet been discovered.

The essential portion of the penicillin molecule, in the words of R. B. Woodward, one of the outstanding organic chemists of our time, was "a diabolical concatenation of reactive groups" that defied all the chemists' most subtle approaches or brutally direct frontal attacks. As we were to discover, a seemingly enchanted ring of chemically active centers, one of them a beta-lactam ring, put the synthesis of penicillin beyond the reach of the most advanced methods available to chemists in the 1940s.

The history of chemical research on penicillin is, by and large, a history of controversy concerning the beta-lactam. The beta-lactam structure was unknown in natural products at the time. A few beta-lactams had been made in the laboratory, but these were well shielded by large groups on the molecule and were not nearly as reactive as the beta-lactam found in penicillins. Therefore, few chemists at the time thought that a beta-lactam could be the heart of the penicillin molecule. Conventional wisdom forbade the presence of the structure and even more forcibly prohibited the presence of a beta-lactam along with other known portions of the penicillin molecule.

The beta-lactam ring is the critical part of the molecule. With that ring structure intact, the molecule possesses antibiotic properties. When the ring is disturbed—and many conditions can disturb it—the desired antibiotic properties disappear. Chemists were faced, therefore, with the difficult problem of working with delicate and reactive groups on the penicillin molecule, groups with which they had had little prior experience, and with chemical tools that were simply too crude for the job. All efforts failed to close the beta-lactam ring or to protect it while performing other chemical operations. At the time of my successful synthesis of penicillin in 1957, I compared the problem of trying to synthesize penicillin by classical methods to that of attempting to repair the mainspring of a fine watch with a blacksmith's anvil, hammer, and tongs.

In contrast to the synthesis program, efforts to master the natural fermentation of penicillin were completely successful. The delicate and chary *Penicillium* mold was coaxed by science and industry into producing more and more precious penicillin. Scientists learned increasingly efficient ways of isolating, concentrating, and purifying the product. The project to elucidate the chemistry of penicillin, however, could boast of far fewer successes. At the end of the wartime penicillin program, penicillin had not been synthesized, and confusion reigned among chemists even about the molecular structure of the compound. After years of study, chemists had accumulated a great deal of information about the chemistry of penicillin; but the more we learned, the more complicated the penicillin problem became.

I was particularly intrigued by the challenge of penicillin synthesis. I had worked with Dr. Max Tishler at Merck & Company in Rahway, New Jersey, on producing streptomycin, and earlier I had studied organic synthesis with Werner Bachmann at the University of Michigan. Perhaps my most important work with Professor Bachmann, while I was a post-doctoral fellow at the University of Michigan, was to develop a commercially feasible synthesis of RDX, the explosive known as cyclonite. Our work, which made large quantities of this high explosive available to the Allies, revolutionized submarine warfare and gave the Allies the advantage at sea. RDX was the explosive that made possible the development of the bazooka and the blockbuster. *Plastique,* as it was known by the French Resistance, changed guerrilla warfare. And so when I met Max Tishler I was already experienced in applying the arcane knowledge of organic syntheses to the solution of real-life problems. Having participated in this work, I was eager to join in the efforts to develop the antibiotics.

Perhaps I was motivated by my vivid recollection of the year I had spent struggling against pneumonia and mastoiditis. That struggle nearly cost me my life. If my doctors had had a course of treatment as effective as that made possible by penicillin, I would probably not have lost that year. As a problem in organic chemistry, moreover, the synthesis of penicillin was a significant challenge. Many had attempted the synthesis. Some had come close; none had succeeded.

Why was the penicillin molecule so difficult to synthesize? Some investigators had believed that the difficulty was due to the source. The lay public and even some professionals believed that because penicillin came originally from a natural source, only living organisms could produce it. We may have difficulty giving this argument much credit today, but such vitalist notions were still current only a few decades ago. And these scientific prejudices occasionally interfered with the rational study of penicillin.

A second difficulty was that old chemical notions interfered with the discovery of new solutions demanded by the penicillin problem. Many prominent chemists doubted that the penicillin molecule could ever be assembled in the laboratory. At one point as many as ninety different structures were proposed for the small penicillin molecule. Eventually, however, the field was narrowed to two: the beta-lactam and the oxazolone-thiazolidine. Evidence mounted in support of a structure for penicillin containing the beta-lactam ring, but no naturally occurring substance was known to contain this structure. The alternative oxazolone-thiazolidine formula was more familiar to chemists. One of the many ironies of the penicillin story is that at least two different reactions to synthesize penicillin that were directed by what turned out to be the wrong formula did actually produce minute quantities of penicillin. On the contrary all efforts to synthesize penicillin by what turned out to be the correct formula proved too difficult and failed.

After studying the results of those early efforts, I reached two conclusions that shaped the course of my own career in chemistry and incidentally changed the course of penicillin research. One was that penicillin was a difficult molecule but, like any other natural substance, could be synthesized by a rational chemical process. The second conclusion was that penicillin could not be synthesized by any combination of techniques known to chemistry at that time. New methods were needed.

My moment of decision was 1948. When I moved from Merck to MIT, I set about devising new methods that would be useful not only in the limited matter of synthesizing penicillin and related compounds but also in solutions to broader synthetic problems encountered in modern organic chemistry and biochemistry.

Many of my friends openly questioned the wisdom of getting involved with penicillin again. The synthesis of that compound was widely considered not only a difficult problem but an elusive one. From the earliest days of the penicillin research, major scientific and technological breakthroughs were continually believed to be just around the corner. But isolation, purification, production, and the chemical identification of penicillin all proved to be inordinately difficult.

Scientific work is ultimately objective; on the way to those ultimate goals, however, scientific work is an art. Intuition, personalities, and luck all play important roles. The laboratory is orderly, the glassware is clean, and the notebooks are pristine and to the point. But the orderly laboratory is a privileged and magical place surrounded by a jungle of disorder. One sympathetic colleague at MIT turned out to be secretly working for a patent adversary. Old friends became acrimonious scientific rivals. Old rivals proved to be surprisingly supportive. In the complicated story of penicillin they all played major roles.

The story of Fleming's stroke of genius is well known. Alexander Fleming had been searching since World War I for antibacterial agents that would kill bacteria selectively without damaging the tissues of the host. In 1928, Fleming found what he was looking for. He noticed that a contaminant in one of his culture dishes was killing the once-thriving colony of staphylococcus bacteria. Fleming accepted this fateful invitation and took up the study of the world's first safe systemic antibiotic. He identified the contaminant as a variety of the mold *Penicillium* and named the antibiotic substance penicillin.

I became involved in penicillin research in a similarly fortuitous manner. After I had been at Merck for about a year, I had some good results to show for my work on calcium pantothenate, streptomycin, vitamin $B_6$, and a few other projects that had turned out rather well. One afternoon Dr. Randolph Major's secretary called me to set up a meeting with the boss. Dr. Major was at that time director of research for the entire group at Merck, not only the chemical division but the microbiological division and others as well. In an administrative sense he was at least two notches higher than I was. I was a group leader. My immediate superior was Dr. Max Tishler, above him was Dr. Joseph Stevens, and then came Dr. Major. So he was considered to be at the top of the scientific pyramid at Merck.

Although I had had some social contact with Dr. Major while at Merck, we had not had much professional contact. I was rather puzzled about why he would want to talk with me.

When I entered his office, Dr. Major said in his characteristically diffident way that he had been noticing from our research reports that I was making rather good progress. He expressed his pleasure.

"You have worked with Professor Bachmann," Dr. Major said to me.

"Yes," I said.

"He is well known for his steroid work," said Dr. Major. Again I said yes, but that I had not done any work with him on steroids. We had had frequent group seminars and so I was familiar with the literature and current work being done on the steroids. But I could not pretend to be an authority.

"Well," said Dr. Major, "we have two problems coming up that we think are going to be important. One has to do with the steroid cortisone. If you would like to work on that problem, I will assign it to you."

When I told Dr. Major that I would feel comfortable working on that problem, he interrupted me to say, "We do, however, have someone coming from Princeton, from

Everett Wallis's laboratory, who has done some work on steroids. His name is Lewis Sarrett."

Dr. Major then went on to say that Merck had decided to work on another interesting problem, namely penicillin. I had heard a little bit about penicillin. I knew that it was supposed to be a remarkable drug but very difficult to work with chemically.

"Yes, that's right," said Dr. Major. "But we think that it is so important we should start on it as soon as we can." He paused for a moment. "So, I will give you your choice. Which one would you like to work on, cortisone or penicillin?"

After a moment I said, "If it is all right with you, Dr. Major, I'll take the penicillin."

Lewis Sarrett eventually synthesized cortisone and later became president of Merck Sharp & Dohme Research Laboratories. I have sometimes joked with him about what would have happened if we had reversed roles. My own guess is that we both would have failed.

Merck had begun developing methods for the production of another antibiotic, streptomycin. Karl Folkers was deeply involved in the research to determine the structure of streptomycin, but he kept running into the problem of purifying the compound for his own research and for general distribution. The drug was produced by fermentation. It was purified by adsorption on charcoal and then elution to remove the material from the carbon. In spite of Folkers's best efforts, most of the streptomycin produced in this way contained impurities that resembled histamine and produced in patients histaminelike allergic reactions—elevated blood pressure, pain, and allergic rashes. Consequently, Merck felt that the streptomycin was still too impure and dangerous for general release.

Max Tishler's group had been working for about six months on the purification of streptomycin. About the same time, my mother had contracted a difficult urinary tract infection. I realized that she was not responding to any of the treatments then attempted and felt that streptomycin might be just the drug she needed. Even though the drug was still in its developmental stages, I thought it was worth the chance. I went to Max Tishler.

Max heard my plea with his usual sympathy and compassion. "Yes, John," he said, "we can make enough streptomycin available to you through our medical department. We can get it to your mother's doctors and see how it works." Then, almost as an afterthought Max said, "You know, John, we've been having a lot of trouble lately in producing pure streptomycin."

"Yes," I said. "I had heard something about the problem."

"Well," Max said, "you know something about this histamine problem. I would appreciate it if you and your group would work on it. The problem is getting very serious."

I asked Max for all the written reports on the histamine problem and for about 100 grams of the impure streptomycin. The reports were impressive. Tishler's and Folkers's groups had tried just about every conventional adsorbent and nearly all the solvents one would normally think of. They even tried chromatography methods. All to no avail. The impurities could not be separated from the streptomycin.

I realized that streptomycin is an amino sugar, very much like cane sugar (sucrose). It is extremely soluble in water, so that I could easily make up a 25 percent solution of streptomycin, just as one could make a sugar solution. The streptomycin solution resembled honey in consistency. I also realized that although amino sugars are soluble in water, they are virtually insoluble in certain organic solvents that are immiscible with water. This extreme solubility in water and insolubility in solvents that do not mix with water struck me as properties worth exploiting in the purification of streptomycin.

Then I remembered an old German process for purifying cane or beet sugar. The major portion of the sugar could be crystallized directly from a concentration of the juice. After removing as much sugar as possible by crystallization, a substantial portion of the impurities remaining in the molasses could be separated from the residual sugar by extraction with liquid phenol. The two problems were similar.

When I mixed phenol and water with the dark brown mixture of streptomycin and its impurities in a separatory funnel, the brown color went almost immediately into the phenol layer. The water layer was clear. I separated the two layers, washed the water layer with ether to remove traces of the phenol, degassed to remove traces of the ether, and then freeze-dried (lyophilized) the remaining product.

Freeze-drying is a slow process. I let it go overnight. In the morning I found the most beautiful colorless solid product at the bottom of the flask. "Now have your people run a test on this," I said to Max. In a few hours, he came running back to say, "That is the best streptomycin we have ever seen."

That problem took me a day to solve. The penicillin problem took nine years.

My friends were probably right in trying to steer me away from penicillin. I had just arrived at MIT, and a young academic chemist is usually dissuaded from undertaking a problem in which his progress is likely to be painfully slow. Because he is bound to be subjected to periodic review by faculty tenure committees, a young chemist is better advised to try dazzling them with a blaze of flashy experiments and a trail of scholarly publications. I settled for a number of smaller victories. There was a whole series of papers with the running title "The Synthesis of Substituted Penicillins and Simpler Structural Analogs" that gave us a lot of running room. We started out with the simple compounds that we could make and gradually worked our way into the more difficult areas of penicillin research.

In all this work, I had one advantage over chemists working in the government-sponsored project during the war. I had, in my view at least, unlimited time. The chemists working on penicillin during the war were under the most severe time constraints. If the program was to continue, successes had to be almost immediate. I decided that I would keep trying until penicillin was synthesized even if I became professor emeritus in the attempt.

My group and I worked out a series of simpler compounds, foothills on the way to the peak. For example, by the time we began our work, the beta-lactam was known to be a key element of the penicillin molecule. By the end of the penicillin project, it was well recognized that the business end of the penicillin contained the baffling beta-lactam ring. Anything that destroyed the ring also destroyed the antibiotic properties of the compound. We made some very simple beta-lactam compounds. This in itself was not much of a trick if one stuck to the older methods. Such beta-lactam rings had been made in the laboratory before. But the older methods had not worked in the synthesis of penicillin. The importance of our early work was that we devised at least four different new methods for making beta-lactam rings under the mild conditions required for a penicillin synthesis.

Once I decided that penicillin was an important problem, and one that had a solution, I never re-evaluated my position. No matter how discouraging the laboratory work turned out to be, I simply went back in and tried more approaches. I went back to the library and read more research reports. I thought more about the problem. As long as I could avoid asking myself the defeating question "Should I really be in this?", I remained immune to the anxieties that accompany scientific research. For me it was always forward march, never halt, never retreat.

Not all scientific projects can be handled in this way. This is certainly not the case in industry, for example. There a research project is reviewed frequently and may be terminated abruptly if the managers of the laboratory feel that

*15   The Lonely Search*

progress is too slow or if they simply decide that it is no longer an interesting or profitable research problem for the company to support. At MIT, on the other hand, I was a research committee of one. I could make the decision to spend the rest of my life on the penicillin problem; it was only my career that was on the line.

I did eventually reach a point when I began to believe that sooner or later we would come up with a rational synthesis of penicillin. During the early 1950s, I was sure that we had developed adequate methods for the delicate synthesis and that the end was in sight. I could not have predicted exactly what methods or materials would be involved in the reactions, but I did begin to feel that these were relatively minor details to be cleaned up. The difficult work of conceiving the general plan of the synthesis and of discovering the singularly appropriate coupling agent for closing the beta-lactam ring had already been accomplished.

It also became apparent in handling the penicillin molecule and some of our simpler analogs that the penicillin structure was not nearly as sensitive as it had been generally believed to be. An inspection of the literature—and I must add my own contributions to that literature as well—emphasized the great sensitivity of penicillin to degradation by acid, base, heat, and other factors. I took few pains to dispel this belief. Certainly it was to my advantage that chemists believe that penicillin was a tough molecule to work with and that anyone working with it should realize that he had a tiger by the tail.

One of the remarkable features of the penicillin work is that there was no competition from the years 1948 to at least 1957. It is essentially unparalleled in modern organic chemistry to have such green pastures entirely to oneself. I had always assumed that I would have lots of competition. The penicillin molecule, after all, had a glamorous history and promised an equally glamorous future.

I once asked R. B. Woodward why I was allowed to approach the penicillin problem all by myself. He said, "John, we all knew that it was in good hands and that you would get it eventually." I believe it is more likely that other chemists were simply tired. They had worked for years on the problem and no amount of talent or money or time could bring them closer to a solution. In fact, it sometimes appeared that the more they knew about penicillin, the farther they moved from understanding it.

# 2 Early History of Penicillin

A curious feature of the history of penicillin is the controversy surrounding its discovery. Alexander Fleming, a bacteriologist working at St. Mary's Hospital in London, shared the Nobel Prize in 1945 with Howard Florey and Ernst Chain, two Oxford scientists, "for the discovery of penicillin and its curative effect in various infectious diseases." But despite the kind words by Professor Liljestrand in introducing Fleming, Florey, and Chain at the award ceremony, partisan arguments about the relative contributions of the three men were thinly camouflaged by the formality of the occasion. The arguments have not abated to this day.

The popular version of the history is an amalgam of the two poles of the debate. People with even the most casual interest in the penicillin story know that the antibiotic was discovered by Fleming. Along with this knowledge, they believe that Fleming made his discovery sometime during World War II. In short, the popular story of penicillin has fused two different aspects of the history of penicillin: the discovery by Fleming and the developmental work done by the group at Oxford ten years later. The heroes themselves, on the other hand, have sought in a variety of ways to resolve the confusion.

When Florey published his own review of penicillin in 1944, he began by claiming flatly that "The chemotherapeutic properties of penicillin were discovered in 1940" (H. W. Florey, "Penicillin: A Survey," *British Medical Journal*, August 5, 1944, pp. 168–171). This became the accepted Oxford view. Fleming, however, had made his critical observation in 1928 and published it in 1929. After the initial work by Fleming, Percival W. Clutterbuck, Reginald Lovell, and Harold Raistrick made several serious attempts at isolating penicillin, but, according to Florey, "the conclusion had been reached that penicillin was an unstable substance and therefore unlikely to have any practical value in medicine."

The Oxford interpretation was promulgated by the influential *British Medical Journal* ("Penicillin: An Antiseptic of Microbic Origin," *British Medical Journal,* August 30, 1941, p. 311). The editors credited Fleming with the discovery of the mold but limited the scope of his scientific contribution to a laboratory technique of perhaps only marginal interest, that is, Fleming's use of penicillin in a differential culture for separating different types of bacteria. Penicillin "does not appear to have been considered [by Fleming] as possibly useful from any other point of view," wrote the editors of the journal. "The wider possibilities of penicillin have been explored at Oxford by a team of workers directed by Prof. H. W. Florey and E. Chain."

Fleming was thus considered by some scientists to be an intruder in a territory controlled by the relative newcomers to the penicillin field, Florey and Chain. John Fulton, professor at Yale Medical School, for instance, wrote to his friend Chester Keefer at the Boston University School of Medicine ( July 7, 1944) that their mutual friend Howard Florey would be passing through Washington on his way from Oxford to Australia.

I might warn you that he seems to be utterly infuriated by the recent account of penicillin in *Time*.... I do not know who gave *Time* its slant. I protested vigorously about it when the editors consulted me prior to publication, but they said that their story had been dictated from the top, and I somehow gained the impression that [Surgeon-General of the Army] Norman Kirk's office must have had a hand in it. I do not personally object to giving Fleming the credit that is his due; but as far as the clinical applications of penicillin are concerned, he had absolutely nothing to do with them. For him, as you well know, penicillin was merely of technical advantage in the culturing of soil organisms. It seems to me that the NRC [National Research Council] should in a quiet way do something to give the American public a little more in the way of proper perspective concerning the most important medical discovery of our time.

A week later, Fulton again wrote to Keefer ( July 14, 1944). Keefer had defended Fleming, albeit weakly, suggesting to Fulton that he reread Fleming's original paper. "The paper, as you say," wrote Fulton, "has a great deal in it, but he [Fleming] did not in 1929 or, as far as I can gather, in any of his subsequent papers, do a single critical experiment that would establish the clinical usefulness of penicillin. . . . It was the type of experiment that Fleming seemed not have the imagination to carry out."

Twelve years after Fleming received the Nobel Prize, his British critics still maintained that he "got a bigger share than he deserved of the credit for penicillin—that the greater part should have gone to Sir Howard Florey and Dr. Ernst Chain, who first took penicillin out of the laboratory and put it into a patient" (*Time*, 1957, vol. 61, p. 60). The Oxford group has consistently pictured their contribution to penicillin as a set of totally new observations going far beyond Fleming's original work. Chain, for example, has written that Fleming did not even recognize the importance of his discovery until the day, eleven years later, when Fleming came to visit Florey's laboratories at Oxford.

In a more charitable gesture, however, before the penicillin boom the Oxford scientists extended a greater measure of credit to Fleming. According to their first paper on penicillin, published in *Lancet* (August 24, 1940, pp. 226–228), Florey and Chain openly acknowledged, "Fleming suggested that the substance [penicillin] might be a useful antiseptic for application to infected wounds." Indeed, in his first report, "On the antibacterial action of cultures of Penicillium, with special reference to their use in the isolation of B. influenzae" (*British Journal of Experimental Pathology*, 1929, vol. 10, pp. 226–236), Fleming wrote the now familiar story of the discovery of penicillin. In 1928 Fleming made a brilliant and deceptively simple observation.

While working with staphylococcus variants a number of culture plates were set aside on the laboratory bench and examined from time to time. In the examinations these plates were necessarily exposed to the air and they became contaminated with various micro-organisms. It was noticed that around a large colony of a contaminating mould the staphylococcus colonies became transparent and were obviously undergoing lysis. Subcultures of this mould were made and experiments conducted with a view to ascertaining something of the properties of the bacteriolytic substance which had evidently been formed in the mould culture and which had diffused into the surrounding medium. It was found that broth in which the mould had been grown at room temperature for one or two weeks had acquired marked inhibitory, bactericidal and bacteriolytic properties to many of the more common pathogenic bacteria.

Fleming was a bacteriologist, not a mycologist. He tentatively identified his contaminant as a strain of *Penicillium rubrum* (Biourge). But he realized the importance of knowing precisely what he had captured on his culture dish. Fleming, therefore, referred the matter to Charles Thom, an American specialist working at the U.S. Department of Agriculture. Thom was just then finishing his book, *The Penicillia* and was the acknowledged expert in the field. Thom positively identified Fleming's strain as *Penicillium notatum* (Westling), a relatively rare *Penicillium* belonging to the group of which *Penicillium chrysogenum* is the type species.

The genius of Fleming was to see a type of phenomenon seen by many others before him and to recognize a new significance in the commonplace and annoying observation that cultures of bacteria occasionally are destroyed by chance contaminants. "To my generation of bacteriologists," Fleming said in his Nobel Lecture, "the inhibition of one microbe by another was commonplace. We were all taught about these inhibitions and indeed it is seldom that an observant clinical bacteriologist can pass a week without seeing in the course of his ordinary work very definite instances of bacterial antagonism. It seems likely that this fact that bacterial antagonisms were so common and well-known hindered rather than helped the initiation of the study of antibiotics as we know it today." However, unlike his professional forebears, Fleming recognized suddenly that the phenomenon that was to be avoided in some contexts could be sought profitably in others. Fleming, and later the Oxford workers, were fortunate in that they hit on an antibiotic that was nontoxic and worked in the human body. If the contaminants could be controlled, they might do important work for the bacteriologist and for the clinician as well.

Ever since serving in World War I as a captain in the medical corps, Fleming had been interested in the destruction of bacteria by leukocytes. "During the 1914–1918 war I spent much time investigating problems in connection with septic wounds, and I was then impressed with the antibacterial power of the leukocytes contained in the pus which exuded from the septic wounds. It was clear from these investigations that the chemical antiseptics in common use were more destructive on the leukocytes than they were on the bacteria" (*British Medical Journal*, 1944). After the war Fleming returned to St. Mary's Hospital Medical School, where he had trained in medicine and had begun research under the great and powerful Sir Almroth Wright. Fleming had been a brilliant student; his academic career showed early promise. In 1919, Fleming was appointed Hunterian professor. He taught bacteriology and investigated bacterial action and the effects of antiseptics. The year of his greatest discovery, penicillin, Fleming was appointed Arris and Gale lecturer at the Royal College of Surgeons.

Fleming's first important discovery was a substance present in tears, mucous secretions, and other natural fluids capable of destroying bacteria. Fleming called this antibacterial substance lysozyme; it is an enzyme capable of lysing bacterial cells. The stories of this important discovery, like stories of the discovery of penicillin, are apocryphal. Sometime in 1922, according to the story, Fleming was at work while suffering from a bad cold. In the course of his observations, he accidentally sneezed on an open culture dish. Later Fleming noticed distinct patches on the plate where the bacteria did not grow. He remembered the sneeze and guessed that some substance in the nasal mucus inhibited the growth of bacteria. Fleming then took a more direct experimental approach to the question. Into a test tube cloudy with a luxuriant growth of bacteria, Fleming dropped some of his nasal mucus. In a short time, the liquid in the test tube was clear, "clear as gin" as Fleming described the effect. The bacteria were dead. Such stories emphasize the ease with which Fleming made scientific progress, a facility that may have had an unfortunate effect on Fleming's reputation as a scientist.

We get a far different impression of Alexander Fleming from his research reports than we get from the Florey and Chain view of the man and his work. The facts contradict Fulton's comment that Fleming "seemed not to have the imagination" for carrying out a critical experiment to establish the clinical usefulness of penicillin. Rather, it seems, Fleming had already demonstrated a talent for the essential observation and the scientific insight for devising a direct course of experiments by which to establish the significance of the observation. Fleming summarized his findings regarding penicillin with scientific precision and with far-ranging imagination.

The toxicity to animals of powerfully antibacterial mould broth filtrates appears to be very low. Twenty c.c. injected intravenously into a rabbit were not more toxic than the same quantity of broth. Half a c.c. injected intraperitoneally into a mouse weighing about 20 gm. induced no toxic symptoms. Constant irrigation of large infected surfaces in man was not accompanied by any toxic symptoms, while irrigation of the human conjunctiva every hour for a day had no irritant effect. *In vitro* penicillin which completely inhibits the growth of staphylococci in a dilution of 1 in 600 does not interfere with leukocyte function to a greater extent than does ordinary broth.

Fleming was not a clinician. He was a bacteriologist. Consequently, his principal interest was in the application of penicillin to the solution of practical problems in bacteriology. A current problem was the study of influenza. In the pandemic of 1918–1919, just a decade before Fleming's penicillin work, an estimated twenty million people died of influenza within a few months. That was the most destructive epidemic in the history of the world, and there was evidence to suggest that influenza might prove to be a recurrent plague.

Epidemiologists and bacteriologists thought at the time that the causative agent was an influenza bacillus *Hemophilus influenzae*. In fact, the disease is caused by a virus that infects the bacteria; but this was not known at the time. Fleming, consequently, was working on what was thought to be a critical aspect of the influenza problem at the time he discovered penicillin. To study the influenza bacillus, bacteriologists needed a reliable means of isolating it without damaging the microbe in the process; hence Fleming's enthusiasm for penicillin as a differential culture medium capable of killing off the penicillin-sensitive microbes and leaving the penicillin-resistant influenza bacillus. Fleming's discovery, furthermore, that perhaps 80 percent of the normal population harbors influenza bacilli without contracting the disease (Fleming and MacLean, "On the occurrence of influenza bacilli in the mouths of normal people," *British Journal of Experimental Pathology*, 1930, vol. 11, pp. 127–134) led Fleming to further studies of the incidence and etiology of influenza. Much of Fleming's original paper on penicillin describes the potential application of the new antibiotic in "the isolation of B. influenzae."

Despite his interest in influenza research, Fleming was not insensitive to the broader possibilities of penicillin. As we have just seen, he tested the toxicity of penicillin broth in animals; he tested the effects of penicillin broth on sensitive tissues of human beings; he observed the effects of penicillin broth on leukocytes; and finally, he irrigated "large infected surfaces in man." All his experiments led him to the conclusion that penicillin "appears to have some advantages over the well-known chemical antiseptics. . . . It is therefore a more powerful inhibitory agent than is carbolic acid and it can be applied to an infected surface undiluted as it is non-irritant and non-toxic. If applied, therefore, on a dressing, it will still be effective even when diluted 800 times which is more than can be said of the chemical antiseptics in use. Experiments in connection with its value in the treatment of pyogenic infections are in progress."

These findings suggested to Fleming that at last he had found the end of his search. As early as 1924 Fleming "was able, by a simple method, to demonstrate clearly the antileukocytic power of antiseptics and to indicate that if the antileukocytic action of an antiseptic was greater than its antibacterial action, such an antiseptic was unlikely to be successful in the treatment of a septic wound" (Fleming, *British Medical Journal,* 1944). When Fleming recognized the action of penicillin, he knew he had found what he sought. Among his summary conclusions, Fleming wrote of penicillin in his original paper: "The action is very marked on the pyogenic cocci and the diphtheria group of bacilli"; "penicillin is non-toxic to animals in enormous doses and is non-irritant; it does not interfere with leukocytic function to a greater degree than does ordinary broth"; and "it is suggested that it may be an efficient antiseptic for application to, or injection into, areas infected with penicillin-sensitive microbes."

Fleming was stung by the squabble over who "discovered" penicillin. He responded to the notice giving Florey and his group full credit for penicillin published in *The British Med-*

*ical Journal.* "It is true," Fleming wrote (*British Medical Journal,* September 13, 1941, p. 386), "that all the work on this substance originated in the accidental contamination of a culture plate with a spore of this *Penicillium.* I think, however, I can claim some merit in the discovery, as without a doubt the same mould has contaminated hundreds of thousands of culture plates and has merely been regarded as a nuisance." Fleming continued, "I do not think that you quite do me justice when you say that, although penicillin was used at St. Mary's and elsewhere as an ingredient of selective media, it 'does not appear to have been considered as possibly useful from any other point of view.'"

Nor was Fleming blind to how penicillin should be developed. He addressed the Pharmaceutical Society (November 14, 1940) on the use of antiseptics in wartime surgery, saying that penicillin would not be used effectively in surgery "until some chemist came along and found out exactly what it was and manufactured it." Fleming offered the opinion at that time that penicillin probably "was quite a simple chemical" and would therefore shortly be in use (*British Medical Journal,* November 23, 1940, pp. 715–716). Fleming spoke from knowledge: ten years earlier Raistrick, Lovell, and Clutterbuck had already begun fundamental studies of the chemistry of penicillin. That their research did not progress quickly discouraged Fleming from the field, but it did not destroy his faith in the effectiveness of penicillin. By 1941, Fleming could be certain of the future penicillin would play. "If its constitution could be ascertained, it would lead to the production of another series of chemotherapeutic agents which may well replace sulphanilamide and its derivatives in medical practice" (*British Medical Journal,* September 13, 1941).

When Fleming first disclosed his observations of penicillin, he had to tread with extreme care. Chemotherapy had not been entirely successful. Paul Ehrlich had spent so much time, earlier in the twentieth century, fruitlessly searching for a "magic bullet" that would annihilate pathogenic cells selectively that most medical authorities were reinforced in their belief that hunting microbes with magic bullets was little more than fantasy. The general medical opinion was, as Fleming's comments reflected, that chemicals are general protoplasmic poisons and always damage the host's tissues to some extent. It had been a general rule of medicine at the time that any substance that is toxic to microorganisms would be toxic to host cells. The commonly accepted alternative was to bolster the natural defenses of the body. Fleming's superior at St. Mary's, the powerful Sir Almroth Wright, moreover, was one of the world-famous proponents of the immunologic approach to the treatment of disease. Fleming may not have been entirely free to make the most of his discovery, and he was also hampered by the nature of his work. He was a bacteriologist working in a clinical setting. He had neither the time nor the resources to develop penicillin fully.

Nevertheless, history and the popular imagination have sided with Fleming in the controversy over who "discovered" penicillin. The person on the street still thinks of Fleming as the discoverer; other workers have fallen into the shadows of history. Florey and Chain are well known to scientists and scholars, but they have not been canonized as Fleming has been. Fleming—El Buen Sabio—for instance, was honored at the yearly fiesta in the fishing village of Gijon, Spain. A photograph of Sir Alexander, larger than life, bore the legend, "To the Holy Virgin we pray: for us, many sardines; for the wizard who gave us penicillin, glory."

The debate about how to assign credit for the discovery of penicillin could not be ignored by the high-minded committee deciding on the award of the Nobel Prize. Opinion was unanimous that the prize for 1945 should be awarded for the development of penicillin. The only question was who to name as the recipient. As late as October 1945—the

Nobel Prize was to be bestowed on December 11—there was strong pressure within the committee and in the larger scientific community to grant a single award to Fleming. Champions of Florey and Chain prevailed on the committee to divide the prize. A tentative compromise was struck by which Fleming would get half the award and Florey and Chain would divide the other half. Finally, controversy was quelled by dividing the prize equally among the three men.

There was an element of chance in the decision by Florey and Chain to begin working on penicillin. Howard Florey had begun to make a name for himself as a new light in physiology and chemistry, bridging the gap between the two disciplines. Ernst Chain was a political refugee, trained primarily as an industrial chemist, and looking for a project after his escape from Hitler's Germany. Chain had originally been funded by a grant from the Cancer Fund, but that support was coming to an end. Florey would need to find another source of money for Chain. The idea of looking at antibacterial substances came from Florey's work with lysozyme. Chain did a few experiments with a visiting American (L. A. Epstein, later L. A. Falk) on penicillin in 1938, but no record of this work is believed to exist. The results were later described by Falk as "not impressive." Norman Heatley, a microbiologist, was asked by Florey to work on penicillin in October 1939. When the war broke out, Heatley had been planning to see Linderstrøm-Lang in Denmark; of course, that plan could not be carried out.

Edward Abraham, an extremely talented biochemist, came into the penicillin research in the spring of 1940 after the first mice experiments had been run. It seemed an urgent matter to purify the substance and to produce enough of it for at least a small-scale clinical trial. Abraham and Chain did this work together. This estimable research team was housed in the William Dunn School of Pathology. A short way up South Parks Road from that laboratory was the equally notable Dyson Perrins laboratories in which Robert Robinson, a brilliant and strong-minded chemist, conducted his own work.

The collaboration of talent from the William Dunn and Dyson Perrins laboratories, which began in 1942, was one of the brilliant periods in British science. But the partnership was not always an easy one, especially when the interactions involved the volatile Ernst Chain. For example, one day toward the end of the collaboration, Chain walked up South Parks Road to discuss the structure of penicillin with Sir Robert Robinson. Chain argued volubly for the beta-lactam structure, which was preferred by Abraham and Wilson Baker; Robinson defended the oxazolone-thiazolidine with equal vigor. Soon the discussion became heated. Robinson rose from behind his desk, seized a bottle of ink, and hurled it at the rapidly retreating figure of Chain. According to accounts of the event, Robinson shouted, "I don't want to see that wretched little man again."

When Chain came to the Sir William Dunn School of Pathology in 1935, his first project with Florey was to look into Fleming's earlier work on lysozyme. Unlike Fleming, Florey was not especially interested in killing bacteria. He had found that lysozyme was also produced as a duodenal secretion and thought that the enzyme might play a role in the pathology of ulcers. Toward the end of their experimental work, Chain and Florey went through the obligatory survey of the scientific literature on lysozyme and other bacteriolytic substances. As a result, Florey and his co-workers found reports of many instances of bacterial antagonism. Among them was Fleming's initial report on penicillin. "This seemed to me a large field, almost completely unstudied," Chain wrote many years later (*TIPS*, 1979, p. 9), "which could bring to light new antibacterial structures of possibly scientific and clinical interest." Florey agreed.

It is clear from a paper he had published with N. E.

Goldsworthy in 1930 ("Some properties of mucus with special reference to its antibacterial functions," *British Journal of Experimental Pathology*, vol. 11, p. 348) that Florey was aware of numerous examples of antibiosis. Indeed, he and Goldsworthy reported several examples they had themselves observed. Chain had claimed that he drew Florey's attention to Fleming's paper, but as Florey was at the time on the editorial board of the *British Journal of Experimental Pathology*, it is inconceivable that he was unaware of it. Furthermore, his colleague at Sheffield, C. G. Paine, had actually used crude penicillin broth to treat eye infections in 1932. What seems to be clear from several sources is that the decision to work on naturally occurring antibacterial substances was arrived at jointly by Florey and Chain (Norman G. Heatley, personal communication).

By a stroke of good fortune, George Dreyer, Florey's predecessor in the chair of pathology at Oxford, had been working on the bacteriophage phenomenon, that is, the infection of certain microbes by parasitic viruses. As experimental organisms for the viruses to infect, Dreyer had used descendants of Fleming's colony of *Penicillium notatum*. (Dreyer died in 1934, but the colony was nevertheless carefully maintained.) The scene was thus set for Florey, Chain, Heatley, and Abraham to begin working on penicillin.

The first problem faced by the Oxford team, as far as penicillin was concerned, was that of learning how to grow the mold. Fleming had used the standard medium of the day—digested bull heart. The Raistrick and Clutterbuck team, working a few years after Fleming, used the classic Czapek-Dox medium of inorganic salts, sucrose, and nitrate. Neither the natural bull heart culture nor the artificial medium, however, was successful. Each kept the *Penicillium* alive but did not coax it to produce more than a pittance of the precious penicillin.

Heatley tried in vain to improve the culture medium by tinkering with the Czapek-Dox recipe. He added glucose, various inorganic salts, and more nitrate, all to no avail. He introduced natural products such as meat extracts, yeasts, malt extract, peptone, glycerol, phosphate, lactate, and thioglycolic acid. He tried changing the concentration of sodium and ammonium ions, oxygen, and carbon dioxide. Regardless of how he altered the nutrient medium, it still took ten days to raise a crop of the mold and several more to purify the meager result. More than 125 gallons of penicillin broth was needed to produce a paltry 200,000 units of still impure penicillin. (The figure 200,000 units may sound like a large quantity of penicillin. The Oxford unit was defined at that time as the amount of penicillin which, when placed in a standard open-ended glass cylinder on a Petri dish containing a culture of penicillin-sensitive bacteria, would produce a bacteria-free zone 25 millimeters in diameter. The large number is the result of mixing scales. The assay is run at a micro level; the production is run at levels orders of magnitude higher. Standard units of penicillin were not set until the late 1940s.)

At first the pinch of muddy brown powder recovered from the isolation process was no more than 1 or 2 percent penicillin. Pure penicillin, as workers would discover years later, is a colorless crystalline substance. Nonetheless, even this tiny yield of penicillin was enough to allow the earliest experimental and clinical investigations of penicillin.

On May 25, 1940, Florey performed his first definitive experiment to demonstrate the possible clinical usefulness of penicillin. He infected laboratory mice with the virulent *Streptococcus pyogenes.* Half the infected mice were left untreated; the other half were given doses of penicillin. After seventeen hours, all the untreated mice were dead. The treated ones were foraging happily in their cages. The experimental findings were dramatic and incontrovertible. There could be no other explanation: the treated mice owed their lives to the therapeutic effects of penicillin.

Florey's next step was to extend his experimentation to

clinical trials. This was a big step, of course. Florey did not know whether human responses to penicillin would be the same as those of laboratory mice. In fact, although Florey was not aware of it at the time, his choice of laboratory animal was fortuitous. He might have chosen guinea pigs and stopped penicillin research on the spot. For reasons that are still not entirely clear, penicillin is toxic to guinea pigs. In experiments with human beings, Florey also faced a serious practical problem: a person would require about 3,000 times the amount of penicillin needed to treat a mouse. Florey also had to find a suitable patient.

Judged by present standards of experimental drug research, the experiment carried out by the Oxford group would be deemed primitive and even legally unacceptable. Working in those blissfully simple times, however, Florey and his group could dispense with the long and expensive process that is now part of the development of any new drug. They never took their research protocol through an Institutional Review Board, nor did they get an informed consent from their experimental subjects. They did not pause for extensive animal testing before going to human subjects. The quick and dirty animal experiment suggested that penicillin was a powerful therapeutic agent. By modern standards the toxicity, even in animals, had not been measured carefully. Florey was indeed fortunate that the crude penicillin and various metabolic by-products contained no seriously toxic substance. If Florey had had to register penicillin as an Investigational New Drug, as pharmaceutical research now requires, the development of penicillin would likely have been delayed by several years and, in fact, might never have become a reality.

Florey's primary contact in the clinical community was Charles M. Fletcher, an Oxford physician at the Radcliffe Infirmary. Fletcher arranged for Florey's first clinical trial of penicillin. The first patient to receive penicillin was a woman dying of breast cancer. She was beyond treatment. No one expected that penicillin would help her. Florey did hope, however, that injecting her with penicillin broth would at least show whether the substance that had so dramatically saved the lives of his experimentally infected mice would be safe for human use. Unfortunately, the penicillin broth did prove to be unsafe. Within an hour, the woman developed a high fever and other signs of untoward reaction to the injected material.

This was a serious setback for penicillin and for Florey's research. Florey and his group had invested their entire supply of penicillin broth in the experiment only to find that the results were sadly negative. Discouraged but not defeated, Florey held doggedly to the conviction that the problem was not with the penicillin itself but with impurities still present in the fermentation broth. Before injecting penicillin broth into another person, it was necessary to find better means of purifying the broth. By good fortune, it was fairly quickly found that the pyrogenic factor was an impurity that could be removed by chromatography on alumina, a process suggested and carried out by Abraham (Norman Heatley, personal communication). Abraham and Chain then prepared a somewhat cleaner dose of penicillin for a second clinical trial.

The second clinical subject was a 43-year-old Oxford policeman, who was also found by Fletcher. The policeman had accidentally scratched himself on the side of his mouth while pruning his roses. The scratch became infected with streptococcus and staphylococcus, and the infection spread to produce suppurating sores all over his body and eventually infected his bones, lungs, and eyes. When he was brought to the attention of Florey, the policeman was near death.

The first treatment was February 12, 1941. Penicillin was in such short supply that it was necessary to recover the drug from the patient's urine for purifying and recycling into the patient. Treatment was continued for five days, during which time the patient improved steadily. Unfortunately, treatment proved to be a Sisyphean task: the team at Oxford could not produce penicillin fast enough to maintain the patient through the complete course of his treatment. Despite his remarkable progress, the patient died.

Florey then made an important tactical decision. Until he had garnered sufficiently large quantities of penicillin, Florey would use his precious penicillin only to treat children. Children, after all, would require significantly smaller doses of the precious drug.

A four-year-old boy suffering from a staphylococcal infection of the face that would surely kill him unless the course of the disease were reversed had a high fever, would not eat, and did not respond to any treatment. After a few days of penicillin treatment, the boy was sitting up in his bed, laughing with the doctors, and eating well. He was clearly on the way to complete recovery when, unexpectedly, he died. Once again the investigators could report scientific success of penicillin but clinical failure. Autopsy revealed, however, that it was not the penicillin that killed the boy but rather side effects of the ravaging staphylococcal infection. The infection had weakened blood vessels in the boy's brain, and he died of a stroke. The most significant autopsy finding, however, was that healing had been well under way.

Despite the boy's death, the treatment proved once again that penicillin was a powerful therapeutic agent in the fight against staphylococcal infection. Florey was thus encouraged to continue the clinical trials. And, indeed, he soon had a series of ten brilliant successes: a fifteen-year-old boy with a streptococcal infection of his hip; a man with a streptococcal carbuncle; a fourteen-year-old boy with a staphylococcal infection of his leg and a secondary kidney infection; a six-month-old baby with a urinary infection; and five patients with eye infections.

Florey reported this series of successful treatments with penicillin in the authoritative British medical journal *Lancet* in 1941. The public beyond the confines of the medical world learned about "the marvelous mold that saves lives" at about the same time from *Time* (1941, vol. 38, pp. 55–56). The *Time* article also warned, however, that penicillin is "difficult and expensive to extract" and that "until it can be synthesized or more cheaply prepared, it will probably only be reserved for desperate cases."

First public disclosure of penicillin research came to the United States from Great Britain and suggested that penicillin research was the exclusive preserve of British scientists. At the time of Florey's clinical trials, however, important penicillin research was already under way in the United States. As early as October 15, 1940, several months before Florey's clinical experiment, Dr. Aaron Alston injected a patient at Columbia-Presbyterian Hospital in New York with penicillin. Another group, led by Dr. Martin Henry Dawson and including Gladys Hobby, microbiologist, and Karl Meyer, chemist, set about producing, extracting, and purifying penicillin in their laboratories at Columbia. Even these experiments were not the first. In 1930 Roger Reid did his doctoral research at Pennsylvania State College to confirm the findings of Fleming and Raistrick. Reid's *Penicillium* cultures were sent to him by Fleming himself. Although Reid could not successfully extract penicillin from the fermentation broth—neither could Raistrick, incidentally—he recognized the importance of the work and kept the cultures intact even after he brought his own research to a close. One early participant in the U.S. penicillin research has described the situation.

When Dr. Florey and his associate, Dr. Heatley, came to this country in the summer of 1941, they visited the few centers at which penicillin was being studied. They also went to the Northern Regional Research Laboratories, at Peoria, Illinois, where arrangements were made for Dr. Heatley to remain for a period. Dr. Florey then visited Dr. Herrell and Dr. Heilman at the Mayo Clinic's laboratories. He was sufficiently impressed with the investigations underway here to give Dr. Herrell 100 mg. of the original Oxford penicillin to be used as a standard in the early work. Dr. Herrell and Dr. Heilman had penicillin isolated [sic] at that time which compared favorably with the penicillin from the Oxford laboratories. Dr. Florey later expressed complete satisfaction with the studies being made here on penicillin [letter from R. D. Mussey, Mayo Clinic, to Ross G. Harrison, chairman of the National Research Council, September 17, 1943].

The age of antibiotics had dawned more or less simultaneously on both sides of the Atlantic.

## Modern Chemotherapy

The modern age of chemotherapy began with the work of Paul Ehrlich around the turn of the twentieth century. This giant of medical science searched for the "magic bullets" with which to chemically combat specific disease-producing organisms. The research of Hans Christian Gram gave him the lead he needed. Gram had earlier discovered that the cell walls of some bacteria would retain specially prepared dyes; others would not. This method of Gram-staining became one of the principal ways of identifying classes of bacteria. It also suggested that different bacteria built their cell walls differently, giving them distinguishing chemical properties.

Ehrlich reasoned that the chemical affinity of the bacterial cell wall and certain dyes might be the basis of selectively destroying bacteria in the body without also destroying the body's own cells. The problem was an easy one to state, but finding the right chemicals with which to destroy selectively cell walls or to interfere with their function was not simple.

Ehrlich's work was prodigious, yet he succeeded in only limited ways. The dye trypan could be used to treat trypanosome infections; a series of arsenic compounds could be used to treat syphilis. But having little chemical theory to guide his search, Ehrlich and other workers in the field were forced to plod systematically through all the organic dyes at their disposal. The work was tedious and often hopeless. According to one story, Ehrlich's antisyphilitic compound Salvarsan was called "606" because he had to investigate that many compounds before finding it.

Throughout his work, Ehrlich found no compound that could be used to treat deep infections. At the turn of the century, any of the common diagnoses was a serious threat to life: scarlet fever, meningitis, rheumatic fever, bacterial endocarditis, osteomyelitis, pneumonia, and septicemia. President Coolidge's son died of septicemia (blood poisoning), the result of a blister raised while he was playing tennis.

Chemotherapy seemed to be a good idea but was beyond the capacity of the best scientists and physicians early in the twentieth century. Immunotherapy, on the other hand, championed by Pasteur in the nineteenth century, was proving successful against a host of diseases. It was, therefore, the treatment of choice among the conservative physicians of the time.

Medical philosophy suddenly changed when Gerhard Domagk, director of research at the Institute of Experimental Pathology of I. G. Farbenindustrie, released his findings on the use of Prontosil to protect mice against experimentally induced staphylococcal infection. Domagk, too, had been driven by the belief that certain organic dyes could be used to kill bacteria. In particular, Domagk worked with the azo compounds. Chemically, azo compounds are characterized by a double bond between two nitrogen atoms; but in the more common experience, they are notable for their intense color—yellow, orange, red, blue, and green.

Gelmo first prepared the azo compound in 1908 and showed that it could be used as a dye. Today about half the dyes used in industry are azo compounds. This would not be the case, however, if Heinrich Hörlein had not succeeded in finding a practical mordant with which to make the new dyes colorfast. In 1909, Hörlein and his co-workers at the Farbenindustrie found that by attaching sulfonamides to the azo compounds, they could produce complex dyes far superior to the simpler azo compounds.

Prontosil, an azo dye.

This compound dye could bind itself very firmly to the protein molecules of wool or silk. Hörlein reasoned that perhaps it would also bind to the protoplasm of bacteria, as Gram's stain had done and, moreover, disrupt the natural function of the protoplasm sufficiently to kill the bacteria. This was indeed the case, and in 1913 it was found that the azo dye chrysoidine had a definite bactericidal effect. A year later, pyridium, a dye closely related to chrysoidine, was in use as a urinary antiseptic. In 1930 another urinary antiseptic, serenium, was also prepared from the azo dye.

On the strength of this long history of research with azo dyes and the application of a few of them to chemotherapy, Gerhard Domagk began a systematic survey of the therapeutic possibilities of all the azo dyes. Two of his co-workers, Josef Klarer and Fritz Mietzsch, synthesized and patented the red dye Prontosil in 1932. (The German patent was not disclosed, however, until 1934.) That same year, Domagk began a series of experiments with mice showing that Prontosil could protect them against streptococcal and staphylococcal infection. In 1933, a ten-month-old baby with staphylococcal septicemia was saved by the use of Prontosil. For this work Domagk received the Nobel Prize in 1938.

Still the question remained: What is the active principle in the red dye Prontosil? The answer was given in 1936 by the team of French chemists, Professor and Madame Trefouel, working at the Pasteur Institute. They split the azo link, separating the colored azo portion of the molecule from the colorless sulfonamide. Their results showed that sulfanilamide—the portion added by Hörlein in 1909 to increase the color binding properties of the azo dye—was the chemotherapeutic moiety of Prontosil.

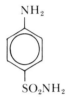

Sulfanilamide.

Suddenly there was great interest in the possibilities of chemotherapy. Colebrook and Kenny (Britain) and Long and Bliss (United States) confirmed Domagk's work. And thus began the hectic activity of producing new derivatives of para-aminobenzenesulfonamide (sulfanilamide) for possible chemotherapeutic applications. In all, about 5,400 compounds were prepared in the decade after Domagk's initial publication, but fewer than twenty were clinically useful. The introduction of the sulfa drugs to the modern pharmacopeia renewed medical interest in chemical means of fighting diseases, but the unfortunately low ratio of successful products to exploratory research dampened enthusiasm somewhat. Thus it was not surprising that when penicillin loomed on the horizon, scientists approached it with mixed feelings.

## Trial of Penicillin under Fire

To the American public, the Cocoanut Grove fire was a bizarre accident. At about ten o'clock one of the patrons of the club decided that he wanted more atmosphere in the already darkened room and broke the light bulb near him. When the bartender noticed this, he told his busboy to replace the bulb. Balancing precariously on a chair and using a lighted match so that he could see the socket, the busboy accidentally set fire to an artificial palm tree nearby. In the mayhem that followed, hundreds of people were trapped in the fire. Heat, noxious fumes, and lack of oxygen killed about a third of the 1,500 people packed into the club.

The devastating fire at the Cocoanut Grove nightclub in Boston on November 28, 1942, gave American civilian, military, and medical authorities what one local newspaper called a "Rehearsal for Possible Blitz" (*Boston Daily Globe,* November 29, 1942, p. 22). Within half an hour of the first fire alarms, the Red Cross had mobilized as if for an enemy bombing raid. The Boston Metropolitan chapter of the Red Cross, supported by twenty local and suburban chapters, had 500 volunteers at their posts. The motor corps commandeered 150 vehicles to be used as ambulances for shuttling victims of the fire from the scene of the disaster to local hospitals. "First aiders," trained in the most modern methods for treating burns and fractures, came into service immediately. It was estimated that at least 300 persons were dead; two days later, at least 500 persons had died (*New York Times*, December 6, 1942, p. 2). Many more would have died if it had not been for the careful use of a new experimental drug, still in its preclinical experimental stages, penicillin.

At the time of the Cocoanut Grove fire, the naturally fermented penicillin was still a closely guarded military secret. Only the scientists and administrators of the Office of Scientific Research and Development, Committee on Medical Research (CMR) knew of the exciting development of the revolutionary new antibiotic derived from a mold. Further, only the most pressing military needs would bring that information out into the open.

The gravity of the situation at the Cocoanut Grove warranted extraordinary responses. Martial law was imposed at 1:35 A.M., and the scene of the fire was cordoned off. Rescue and treatment became a military operation.

Joseph M. Laughlin, regional manager of the First Civilian Defense Area exercised his authority under the extraordinary wartime powers granted him to release the precious store of plasma and other emergency medical supplies held in readiness should German bombers attack Boston. The city's hospitals were put on emergency alert. Air raid rescue crews were mobilized. Never before had such large-scale medical resources been organized. It was, said Laughlin, "an epic in medical history" (*Boston Herald,* December 1, 1942, p. 1). He spoke more than he knew.

To the military medical authorities, under the direction of the CMR, the fire was also a natural laboratory in which to learn how best to prepare for the acute traumas that accompany combat. Doctors N. W. Faxon (director) and E. D. Churchill (chief) of the West Surgical Service of Massachusetts General Hospital were put in charge of the natural experiment, treating about 40 of the victims with the most modern methods then available; the remaining 180 treatable victims were taken to Boston City Hospital.

Treatment of the fire victims became a major news item, especially after the CMR attempted to keep the lid on the story. The general public was told "that no new treatments have been applied" (*Boston Globe,* December 1, 1942) or were contemplated in coping with the massive burns and pneumonias resulting from the inhalation of hot air, smoke, and noxious fumes. The accepted treatment for massive burns was to coat the victim with ointments—especially Sperti-bio-deyne—or with tannic acid. No treatment, however, was capable of preventing the infections that inevitably followed.

An urgent order was put through to Merck, kept under the strictest secrecy, for any of the miracle drug—penicillin—that they could spare. The CMR made the quick decision to release penicillin. I was working at Merck at the time. When we received the order at Merck, various groups, including Max Tishler's, of which I was a member, went to work concentrating and purifying the crude penicillin broth. We worked around the clock, in relays, and within a short time had concentrated and purified all the crude fermented penicillin we could obtain. With the same urgency, we prepared the product for shipment to Boston.

"Police escorts from four states accompanied a consignment of an as yet unnamed drug rushed to the Massachusetts General Hospital early this morning from the Merck & Co., Inc. Laboratory in Rahway, N.J. for treatment of fire victims," reported the *Boston Globe* (December 2, 1942, p. 15). The report continued, "A 32-liter supply of this drug, described as priceless by a laboratory technician, will be used to prevent infection from burns. The mercy vehicle arrived at 4:30 this morning, after a seven-hour, 368-mile drive through steady rain."

Supplies of penicillin were severely limited. In the Merck laboratories as well as in the laboratories of the other major companies, every milligram of penicillin was jealously hoarded. Penicillin went for treatment and clinical experiments, not primarily for chemical research. Dr. Max Tishler once responded to a laboratory technician's request for something more than the pitifully small dole of penicillin we were allotted for research. "Remember," said Max Tishler, "when you are working with those 50 or 100 milligrams of penicillin, you are working with a human life."

The wonder drug was finally out in the open world. "There was some discussion of requests for publicity with respect to penicillin," Keefer reported to the CMR (minutes,

December 3, 1942), "and the Committee decided that the time was not yet ripe for publicity." Once the news media realized what penicillin was, however, it became increasingly difficult to force the genie back into the lamp.

The trial under fire at the Cocoanut Grove demonstrated just how true those words were. John Fulton wrote to Ross G. Harrison (October 4, 1944) about the spirit of the times when penicillin research was still in its earliest, most difficult stages. "Some of our friends pooh-poohed Florey when he came over in July 1941, and you are the only one so far as I am aware who envisaged the possibilities. Even the Rockefeller Foundation felt that Dan O'Brien was crazy for having sponsored the trip; but now you might think that they had discovered penicillin themselves!"

# 3 Developing the Secret Weapon

Penicillin research was classified as SECRET in 1942. At that time, before the proliferation of military security classifications, SECRET was a strict military marking. Records had to be stored in a steel safe with a three-tumbler lock. Any records to be destroyed had to be burned in the presence of a specially designated official who would attest to their appropriate and complete destruction. The officer took responsibility for the destruction by signing a special notebook kept for the purpose. He was legally liable.

For scientific or commercial research to be subjected to such tight security was unusual. Reasons for the secrecy, however, were a complex web of military, diplomatic, scientific, and proprietary interests. I will have to digress from the main line of my story about the scientific development of penicillin to sketch in some details of that social and political history. To the best of my knowledge, this story has never been told.

## The Beginning of Government Involvement in Penicillin Research

On June 28, 1941, President Roosevelt signed Executive Order No. 8807 establishing the Office of Scientific Research and Development (OSRD). Extraordinary powers had been granted him a month earlier for coping with the "unlimited national emergency" of possible war with Germany and Japan. The OSRD was given charge of "assuring adequate provision for research on scientific and medical problems relating to the national defense." Dr. Vannevar Bush was appointed director.

President Roosevelt and Vannevar Bush felt that the nation's medical and scientific talent should be better organized and consolidated during a time of war. As a result, they brought together a select group of men, drawn from the forty-two scientific and advisory committees and councils already under the aegis of the National Research Council and formed the OSRD Committee on Medical Research (CMR): Dr. A. Newton Richards (chairman of the CMR and vice president in charge of medical affairs at the University of Pennsylvania), Dr. Lewis H. Weed (Johns Hopkins), Dr. A. R. Dochez (Columbia), Dr. A. Baird Hastings (Harvard), Brigadier General James Stevens Simmons, Rear Admiral Harold W. Smith, Dr. L. R. Thompson (U.S. Public Health Service).

At the first meeting of the CMR, Bush outlined his expectations of how the committee would function: "He would look to the Committee on Medical Research for its independent judgment, which he would not in any way attempt to influence" (CMR minutes, July 31, 1941). The CMR would initiate new research programs, involve itself in defense activities, and establish a liaison with the British in all areas pertaining to military medicine. As the CMR matured and gained influence, the committee became the political arm of the research establishment already in place at the National Research Council.

Men on the committee were all familiar with the Washington bureaucracy. They had come up through the ranks of the National Research Council and were at home with the push and shove of politics. They knew how to establish a large and effective organization, how to manage people and information, and above all, how to keep the wheels of the organization moving. The lubricant, relatively abundant as Washington mobilized for war, was money. At the end of July 1941, the Committee of the Bureau of the Budget transferred to the OSRD account $1,170,000, "to be expended upon medical research." Of this sum, $1 million was to be spent for work done under contracts; $170,000 was for "administrative expenses" (CMR minutes, July 31, 1941). There was also a tacit promise of virtually unlimited funds for whatever medical research programs might aid in the war effort.

One week after the CMR first convened, the committee discussed "the futility of trying to get anywhere on one million dollars" (CMR minutes, August 7, 1941). Chairman Richards responded by saying that Director Bush had anticipated their complaints by submitting a request to the Budget Committee of Congress for an additional $17 million, of which at least $4 million would go directly to the CMR. But Richards also reminded the committee, "We can't go to Congress, and he [Bush] can't say, 'Give me $25,000,000 for medical research.' We must have some budget which can be defended." Richards was cautious but continued, "I don't think it is necessary to be too pessimistic about funds" (CMR minutes, August 7, 1941). Richards was right.

The first order of business for the new committee was to decide on a course of action that deftly balanced the research interests of the medical people and the pragmatic needs of the military people. Compromise was difficult from the outset. Admiral Smith, for instance, argued that "military medical services operated within the limits of military efficiency" (CMR minutes, August 7, 1941). The goal of saving lives was not in itself sufficient. To be approved by the committee, therefore, the medical expertise gained as a result of a program sponsored by the CMR had to demonstrably enhance the military position of the Allies.

The committee reviewed military medical experience gathered during World War I for what it might teach about the demands of the more modern conflict. From this review came the initial projects of the CMR: mechanical protection of the soldiers' chest and abdomen by means of carefully designed protective clothing and armaments; dressing wounds and burns; extensive clinical study of the sulfa drugs to determine the most effective ways of using them in the field; treatment of shock and other traumatic effects of sudden loss of blood after severe battle wounds; the development of suitable blood extenders or substitutes; control of tropical disease by means of antimalarial drugs and insecticides.

The most difficult decision the committee had to face concerned penicillin. Florey's published reports of clinical miracles wrought by penicillin were exciting, but many problems remained to be solved before penicillin could be a useful drug. In addition to the routine difficulties of medical and scientific research, the CMR had the extreme pressure of time. After all, it was not an academic or commercial development laboratory. According to the mandate from Congress, the CMR would function only as long as the military situation required. The committee was an emergency wartime agency of the government, created to promote the war effort. When the war effort no longer required such an agency, the CMR would be dissolved.

The amount of information accumulated about penicillin during the period from 1928 to 1941 was distressingly small. The pioneers, taking their lead from Fleming in the early 1930s, had found that a salt of penicillin was soluble in water and in alcohol but was not soluble in the organic solvents ether or chloroform. They also devised a synthetic medium on which the *Penicillium* could be fermented without adversely affecting the antibiotic properties of the penicillin it produced. They found a way of extracting penicillin—at least in an impure and amorphous state. At the same time, however, chemists recognized with growing alarm that acids, bases, oxidants, and other factors could apparently destroy the antibiotic properties of the molecule. This was the sum of knowledge about penicillin; and all the information about penicillin showed that it was a difficult substance to work with.

The prudent men of the CMR were justifiably wary of getting involved in such an open-ended research program. Even as late as December 1942 Richards commented on "the speculative character of the whole penicillin enterprise" (letter from Richards to M. Demerec, December 1942). But "chimerical as [penicillin] was regarded in certain quarters" (Baxter, 1968, p. 346), the CMR was "an ardent and steadfast exponent" of the penicillin program.

Nevertheless, within a year of Perrin H. Long's initial inquiries about penicillin, the committee resolved formally "that the Chairman be authorized to suggest to interested persons the desirability of a concerted program of research on penicillin involving the pooling of information and results" (CMR minutes, October 2, 1941).

In its first year of operation, the CMR did not invest much of its $1.6 million budget in pure research. Ten small studies of adrenal and other steroids were undertaken in the belief that directly administering these hormones, mobilized normally by the body in time of stress, could prevent fatigue and heighten responsiveness. The other eighty-six contracts awarded by the CMR that first year were to develop protective clothing, treatment of shock and injury, and rehabilitation of the wounded. According to the minutes, the only expenditure on penicillin during the period ending February 15, 1942, was $8,250 to Robert D. Coghill at the Northern Regional Research Laboratory in Peoria, Illinois, for work on the natural fermentation of penicillin. From this small beginning, the CMR grew to be a major influence on the course of medical science in the United States. It granted a total of 600 contracts at 133 universities, research foundations, and commercial laboratories. A staff of 1,500 professionals, M.D.s, Ph.D.s, and 4,000 support staff was organized. The total expenditure has been estimated at about $24 million (Baxter, 1968, p. 300), although I suspect that it was higher.

The CMR had a difficult mission with respect to penicillin. It not only had to initiate research programs in the national interest, administer them, and ultimately oversee the practical applications of their fruitful research but maintain a delicate balance of commercial interests and public concerns. This control would eventually mean that the committee would be responsible for "organizing and promoting research on the synthesis of Penicillin," financing the research projects at various commercial and academic laboratories, arranging for the exchange of information about the synthesis problem, working out with the firms involved in the program "equitable arrangements concerning patents," conducting all nonmilitary clinical research, distributing penicillin, and dealing with representatives of the Allied governments "in regard to disclosure of information relating to research on synthesis" (memo of CMR meeting on the penicillin program, August 31, 1943).

The CMR decided early in the program that production of the natural penicillins would be left to the commercial firms and that the more speculative research into the structure and possible chemical synthesis of penicillin would remain under the strict control of the OSRD. As much as possible, the synthesis program was to be kept separate from the fermentation program. Although the expense of parallel programs would be great, gearing up for a penicillin industry based on the naturally fermented product would at least assure a supply of penicillin. The synthesis program was a much greater risk because so little was known about the chemistry of penicillin at the time.

Richards and Bush recognized the simple truth that the commercial interests would not develop penicillin unless they were guaranteed some enjoyment of the fruits of their labors and investment. Somehow the companies that participated in the development of penicillin had to be permitted exclusive rights to their discoveries. Once the research and development of penicillin were completed, no one could be allowed to jump on the penicillin bandwagon for a free ride. The CMR thus found itself in the awkward position of needing to devise a system by which private companies would gain patent rights to processes and products developed, at least in part, with public money. The CMR would coordinate the research and development activities of the several interested commercial firms and, at the same time, would direct the research activities of the public and non-profit organizations in such a way that their findings would be made available to all legitimate parties to the agreement. Such an arrangement required that the private firms waive some of their usual proprietary rights in the development of a potentially useful and lucrative product. The special arrangement also required the selfless cooperation of many government scientists who would not gain personally from the success of the penicillin program.

In establishing the rules for working on penicillin, the CMR tried mightily to avoid conflicts of private and public interests. Legal departments in the government and in the pharmaceutical companies worked for years on the formalities of the agreements to investigate penicillin and produce it. The agreements were so difficult, in fact, that the final wording was not hammered out until after the government had suspended the project.

In contrast to the bureaucrats, the scientists had to show results immediately. "I remember Heatley's coming to Merck well," said Karl Folkers. "The day after, we got a carpenter in and Bob Peck had some steps built, some wooden steps, so that he could stand on these steps and pour solvent solutions on the top of a great big chromatographic column, because chromatography was going to be the key step in purification. Bob calculated that he wanted a big column, and he couldn't reach the top of the column without some wooden steps. And so in effect we started getting geared up to do penicillin the very next day. There was no hesitation, no arm-twisting, no persuasion, no nothing. The next day, we were in business gearing up to work on penicillin."

Robert Coghill of the Northern Regional Research Laboratory (Peoria, Illinois) was sent on a site visit by the CMR and saw those steps just after they were built. "Merck has a very beautiful set-up for the continuous extraction of penicillin from 1,000 liters of culture fluid per week," he reported to the CMR. "They apparently really mean business in this penicillin work as they have plans drawn and are acquiring apparatus to process ten times this amount of material" (CMR minutes, December 31, 1941).

### International Cooperation and Intrigue

Full-scale cooperation between the United States and Great Britain on the penicillin project was officially established in 1942. A year before that time, however, a special envoy came from Great Britain to the United States to enlist support for such a joint research and development venture. Howard Florey and Norman Heatley left Great Britain for the United States on June 26, 1941, on a secret mission to involve American scientists and manufacturers in penicillin research and, should luck favor their work, mass production of the antibiotic.

At that time, Great Britain was already at war with the armed forces of the Third Reich. Hitler's *blitzkrieg* had subdued Poland and most of western Europe. The massive retreat of the British Expeditionary Forces from the beaches of Dunkirk had already taken place a year before. Italy had entered the war. The British had staged their counteroffensives in the bitter North African campaigns, but the future of the war looked bleak to the British. Florey described the situation: "The first human patients were treated in the winter of 1940–41, at the time of the worst enemy bombing of England. It seemed improbable that much headway could be made in getting large-scale production started in this country" (H. W. Florey, "Penicillin: A Survey," *British Medical Journal,* August 5, 1944, pp. 168–171). In the United States, on the other hand, hope still triumphed over experience: although the engines of war were being cranked up for action, the United States was not yet formally at war with the Axis powers. Edward Abraham has described Florey's position:

If one were thinking of getting penicillin produced and used in war medicine, we had no option. I think Florey's decision was the right one, to go to the United States, because first of all, this country was being subjected to heavy bombing and there was considerable disorganization. Everything had to have a priority. Penicillin had some priority, but it had to compete with a lot of other things. Second, I have the feeling that some aspects of the fermentation industry were better run in the United States than they were here. I may be wrong in that, but one of the first major advances in production made in the United States was the use of deep fermentation and the discovery of the use of precursors. To my knowledge, there was nothing in Europe, with the possible exception of citric acid and alcohol, of course, to compare with the deep fermentation methods that were being worked out in the United States.

In its early stages, the Anglo-American cooperation in penicillin research was no secret. The latest findings and joint ventures were publicized in the popular press as an outstanding instance of Allied solidarity in the face of Axis threats to peace and security. They were also promoted as examples of democracy at work: the willing cooperation of free scientists, industrialists, and government agencies in the struggle to solve complex scientific and technological problems in the effort to improve the lot of humankind. The motives behind the massive program to domesticate *Penicillium* and to eventually synthesize penicillin were thus a rich mixture of propaganda, scientific advancement, and commercial opportunism.

The binding energy that brought these three disparate interests together and maintained them, however, was friendship and the war. Florey said that he was not at all sure that this would have come off at all had it not been for his earlier friendship with Richards, because they knew each other, trusted each other, and Richards took some notice of what he said (Abraham transcript). As a result, Florey immediately had the ear of the CMR, of which Richards was chairman, and of Merck, where Richards sat on the Board of Directors. Florey later told one of his colleagues, "It was then that my former acquaintanceship with A. N. Richards paid off, because it turned out that it was possible to persuade the American government to put substantial sums of money into penicillin production via the pharmaceutical industry."

The scientific mission by Florey and Heatley was only the first of several exchanges of information and personnel between the two countries. John R. Mote, deputy director of the British Ministry of Supply, wrote to Richards (December 21, 1942) to enlist the help of the United States in the "urgent efforts" to raise the production of penicillin in Great Britain. "We are informed that a new method of production has been or is being evolved," he wrote (OSRD CMR general file). Mote asked that two research scientists from the Wellcome Research Laboratories, Drs. Trevan and Pope, be allowed to tour United States penicillin plants. At the bottom of Mote's letter, Richards made the note, "Full disclosure promised by both Merck and Squibb. Notified by phone. Dec. 31. A.N.R."

Soon after this exchange, the British sent their highest level administrator-scientists to a meeting with the CMR. Sir Henry Dale, president of the Royal Society of London and member of the Medical Research Council, and Dr. E. D. Adrian, professor of physiology at Cambridge, attended the meeting and called for a discussion of "the status of research on certain medical aspects of defense in England" (CMR minutes, January 8, 1942).

Correspondence between the research laboratories on either side of the Atlantic was carried in the British and American diplomatic pouches. One of the earlier reports of an improved method for preparing penicillamine, which was discovered by the Oxford group, for instance, came in this way. The contents were made available to us at Merck late one Friday, and I worked on the method all through the weekend with Max Tishler and others. Max had developed the team approach to important research problems, keeping the laboratories in action day and night until the problem was solved. On Monday, we scheduled a meeting with the other participants in the American side of the penicillin program. At that meeting the question was casually raised as to whether someone should try to duplicate the important work reported by the Oxford group. Max Tishler and the other Merck workers held their peace; but we all knew that several hundred grams of penicillamine had already been prepared and was available in the Merck laboratories. This was typical of the way Merck operated at that time.

The CMR had taken the position from the very first that "in general the Committee on Medical Research would avoid publicity" (CMR minutes, July 31, 1941). Beyond this, members of the committee also recognized "that conferences starting out in open problems might soon turn to matters of a confidential or secret character" (CMR minutes, July 31, 1941). As a result, the committee decided that clearance of all consultants and other scientific personnel in sensitive positions in the penicillin program would be essential.

Military needs for secrecy often took precedence over the need for open scientific communication in the penicillin program. Major General James G. Magee, Army surgeon general, informed Harvey H. Bundy, Office of the Secretary of War (June 20, 1942), that neither international treaties nor the accepted rules of war allow for any distinction between friendly and enemy wounded personnel. "It would be shortsighted, however," Magee said, "to fail to recognize that knowledge in certain fields of medical science may bear more directly on the military situation than on the welfare of the individual." Magee was therefore against communicating penicillin information too widely. "The free dissemination of such information can be of very material aid to the enemy. It, therefore, becomes an instrument of warfare and its publication on the grounds of humanitarianism cannot be justified."

General Magee recommended strict censorship of all penicillin correspondence. He was not alone in proposing this drastic wartime measure. Although censorship went against the grain of scientists, accustomed as we were to the free exchange of basic scientific knowledge, and offended the civil libertarians in the government, strict control of the penicillin information became a prerequisite of the penicillin program itself.

Occasionally the security imposed major scientific inconveniences. "We get a tremendous number of documents from England and Canada," complained one CMR member. "The difficulty is only that most of them come labeled with a British designation SECRET AND CONFIDENTIAL, and it is impossible to circulate those widely" (Dr. Lewis Weed, CMR minutes, August 7, 1941). When Florey was asked about the degree of British secrecy imposed, "he was very much surprised that it was held SECRET AND CONFIDENTIAL in Washington" (Dr. Cannon, CMR minutes, August 7, 1941). Great Britain and the United States were clearly getting their signals mixed; and, as a result, the penicillin program suffered and would continue to suffer unless something was done.

To resolve the confusion, "a code of quasi censorship rules" (CMR minutes, July 3, 1942) was drawn up by which to regulate all communications on penicillin. At first by informal agreement all penicillin information was passed through the CMR. Richards suggested to Coghill that "I should be glad to have you consider the propriety of the distribution of that information through this Committee." When Coghill was to give a popular talk on "the history of penicillin" to the Washington Rotary Club, Coghill had to ask Richards to clear the information. Richards responded, "I am not worrying about what you will say concerning penicillin, confident, of course, that you will say nothing whatever about the chemistry of the substance or the advances which are being made" (November 13, 1943).

The British established similar censorship regulations. The British Medical Research Council controlled all communications about penicillin. Unfortunately, confusion still arose between the British and the American censoring agencies. Sir Henry Dale wrote to Richards (November 5, 1942) about the matter, "which gives me some concern and I wish we had had a full-dress discussion of it with you and your colleagues when I was over." Sir Henry continued,

It seems to me that judgments on our two sides of the Atlantic on the question of secrecy with regard to new therapeutic or prophylactic knowledge are capricious and inconsistent and that the authorities dealing with the matter have no agreed or intelligible principles of action. One set of observations made here were suppressed for some 1½ years until the same began to be published openly by workers on your side who knew nothing of what our men had done. Now colleagues of mine wish to publish in another field and . . . we hear that your side will not publish such matter and hope that we won't. I wish that you would try to get a clear statement of principles. Personally I am against all this suppression and want the Red-X over research.

In June 1942, the CMR instructed the chairman of the Censorship Committee to draw up a statement of censorship principles. This he did, but throughout the penicillin program, the issue of censorship and suppression of scientific information galled the scientists involved.

Why was such censorship imposed? I think that there were two reasons for the secrecy: international espionage in time of war was a very real possibility; and industrial espionage was as likely then as it is at any time.

Early in the war, Florey realized that Germany and Japan might be interested in penicillin. He wrote to Sir Edward Mellanby of the Medical Research Council, saying that it seemed "very undesirable" to him that cultures of penicillin or information about current penicillin research should be broadcast widely, lest "it should go to the Germans" (quoted in Bickel, 1972, p. 133). Florey therefore gave instructions that the National Type Collection Laboratories not issue samples of penicillin or related materials "to anyone with possible enemy connections."

In the United States the CMR had similar concerns. The minutes for November 23, 1944, record a discussion about sending samples of penicillin to the Pasteur Institute. "In view of the possible leaking of such information to the enemy, the Committee took no action . . . pending the receipt of additional information."

Fear that the enemy would learn about penicillin research was widespread. In 1943 two pharmaceutical firms operating in the United States, Hoffman-LaRoche and CIBA, expressed their eagerness to enter the penicillin program. Richards was informed by his assistant Carroll L. Wilson, however, that participation by these two companies was not a good idea. "These companies are of foreign ownership and under foreign management," Wilson said, "and although they may be fine, high-minded groups, nevertheless, it might be well to go slowly in furnishing them information on deep fermentation culture or synthesis" (September 4, 1943, OSRD Director's Special Subjects Correspondence file [Dir. Spec. Subj. Corres. file]).

The belief was widespread that both the Germans and the Japanese would develop a penicillin industry. They certainly had the prerequisites. Both nations had well-developed fermentation industries in operation: the German beer production and the Japanese soy and sake industries. Both nations had put great emphasis on technological advance. The Germans, moreover, had the resources of the vast and experienced I. G. Farbenindustrie and a long tradition of outstanding advancements in organic chemistry at both the academic and industrial levels. Finally, German and Japanese scientists had ready access to the open literature on penicillin before the war. Why, then, did neither country develop a penicillin industry during the war?

German intelligence in Sweden monitored Florey's reports of his clinical trials of penicillin (reported in *Lancet,* August 1941) and sent them immediately to Heinz Oppinger. Oppinger was the most likely recipient of those intelligence reports because he had been the first German biochemist to attempt the identification of a penicillin-yielding mold. He was the first to work on the extraction of the active principle in penicillin (Bickel, 1972, p. 296). He had worked for two years as assistant to Hans Fischer in Munich and had managed to extract a small amount of penicillin at his laboratory in the Hoechst Chemical Company.

Oppinger's work did not progress quickly, and when the German military-medical authorities tried to enlist the support of the extensive German pharmaceutical and chemical industries in a penicillin program in late 1943 they encountered so much resistance that their projects fell through. Much later, Bayer (Leverkusen), Schering (Berlin), and several university research groups did become interested in penicillin. But by then it was too late for a German program. The war had turned against the Germans who, by this time, were desperately fighting for the survival of the Third Reich.

The Germans did not fail to recognize the propaganda value of penicillin, however. Early in 1944, Hitler awarded the Iron Cross to his personal physician, Theodor Morrell, for his discovery of penicillin. This was a patently false accolade.

Hamilton Southworth, an American intelligence agent, toured Europe collecting military-medical intelligence during the war. In his *London Newsletter* (No. 103, September 2, 1944) to the intelligence authorities in Washington, Southworth wrote, "Nitti and Trefouel have the Fleming strain, number 4222, of *Penicillium notatum* and produce penicillin by surface culture and amyl acetate extraction, with or without carbon adsorption. The process has been turned over to Rhone-Poulenc but the total output is only about 400,000 units per week. . . . No work has been done on the chemistry of penicillin." In the same dispatch, Southworth reported on what meager evidence we could find for a German penicillin effort. "We found no evidence that the Germans were actually producing penicillin. About 8 months ago, they tried to obtain the Fleming strain from the Institut Pasteur but were alleged to have been given a false one. Later they said they were organizing their own program, but as recently as last June [1944], Schlossberger was searching for an active strain."

A year later the war was over and Southworth visited the laboratories at Elberfeld-Leverkusen. He reported that "Penicillin—Experimentation with Penicillin was about where we were 2 to 3 years ago. Weyland showed the laboratory where it is made on a 2-gallon scale, the best concentration yet achieved being 2000 [*sic*] units per milligram. Some efforts directed at deep culture production were underway. No chemical analysis has been possible."

The most probable explanation for the German failure to develop a penicillin industry was their reliance on the familiar sulfa drugs. Much of the early work on sulfa drugs had been done in Germany, and, presumably, German scientists felt that sulfa would be the drug of choice. They discovered penicillin too late.

The situation in Japan may have been different. Like the

Germans, the Japanese tried at the last moment to develop a penicillin industry. Japanese scientists were informed of the German developments in penicillin, and in June 1944, Japan sent a submarine to Hamburg, where the Japanese military attaché stationed in Berlin transferred to the ship German and British scientific reports. A dried sample of the mold was also sent back to Japan. Hamao Umezawa, Director of the Institute for Microbial Chemistry in Tokyo, has described the situation.

In November 1943 I was working in the medical school of Tokyo University and also in a section of the Army Medical School, where it was our responsibility to plan basic research. At that time, I knew that important foreign scientific journals had suddenly appeared in the Army Medical School library. They had been carried by Japanese submarine from Hamburg, probably, to Japan sometime in July or August of 1943; and they carried reports of the latest research in medicine and weapons.

Among those journals, in *Klinische Wochenschrift* for 1943, I found very interesting articles on penicillin and other antimicrobial compounds produced by microorganisms. One article in particular, written by Dr. Kiese, reviewed the penicillin studies then going on in England.

Because the section to which I belonged had the responsibility of finding a good subject for research, we decided to propose penicillin for the study. As part of my effort to convince the Army Medical School, I translated the Kiese article into Japanese at the end of 1943 and circulated it among my colleagues. Other investigators saw the possible value of penicillin, so that very quickly we organized joint research groups.

We first investigated a fungus strain that must have been wrongly classified because, although it was classified as *Penicillium notatum,* it did not produce any antibiotic compounds. The pigment produced by that strain was more green than the yellow pigment we were led to expect from our reading. At the end of January 1944, I believe it was 27 January 1944, the Asahi newspaper began printing a series of reports from Buenos Aires on penicillin research in England and in the United States. Most of the reports were of English research. At one point, for instance, it was reported that Winston Churchill was suffering from pneumonia and that penicillin treatment cured him in four days. The information was wrong, we later learned. Churchill was treated with sulfathiazine; doctors were reluctant to treat him with the new penicillin drug.

This series of articles stimulated the Army Medical School to begin penicillin research. I was called by Major Inagaki to request a meeting of the experts in fungus research, biochemistry, pharmaceutical chemistry, and fermentation. Two days later, we had our meeting; the most famous investigators in Japan came together. . . .

The joint study proceeded well until June 1944. After that, the temperature became higher than 25°C. That is the reason why after that no progress was made. In July, I moved as Assistant Professor to the Institute for Infectious Diseases of Tokyo University. I waited until the beginning of September. We then selected many culture filtrates. Two of them produced a golden yellow pigment in a milk medium. Those cultures also produced active compounds against staphylococcus but not against E. coli. Ultimately, these cultures were not selected for further research.

However, one culture grown on my desk, where the temperature was just right, was found to inhibit bacteria. The ether extract inhibited the growth of staphylococcus, even when diluted by 1 million.

My brother, who was then at the Fujiwara Institute of Technology (later transferred to Keio University), concentrated the filtrate, transferred it to water, treated with barium carbonate, and obtained a beautiful precipitate. When he analyzed this precipitate, the result was exactly the same as that reported by Dr. Heilbron in the review article by Dr. Kiese. We were certain, therefore, that the compound we had isolated must have been penicillin. It inhibited staphylococcus at a dilution of 6.4 million.

I reported this in the monthly meeting of the Institute for Infectious Diseases, November 1944. My brother reported his results in December 1944 to the Japanese Chemical Society in Tokyo. The Army Medical School then asked the Morinaga Confectionary Company near Hakone to begin penicillin production. The next day, Dr. Iwadari and his father appeared in my laboratory. He was assistant professor at Tokyo University at that time. They said that the Banyu Pharmaceutical Company could make incubator rooms in the factory. I therefore gave them two strains of our penicillin. In February or March, I was asked to visit Dr. Iwadari's factory. He had arranged a human chain to perform all the mechanical operations of mixing, shaking, separating, and purifying the penicillin from the fermentation broth. Thirty or forty women stood in a long row at tables, adding the proper reagents, shaking the bottles, and then passing them on to the next woman in the chain. The system worked, and before the end of the war, the Morinaga Company and the Banyu Company were supplying penicillin to the Army Medical School.

In November 1944, Japanese scientists announced that they had established a large-scale production plant (*New York Times,* November 17, 1944, vol. 12, p. 4). This report, like the earlier German one, was little more than propaganda.

### The British Come to Peoria

When Florey and Heatley left Great Britain for the United States, enthusiasm for penicillin in England was not high. In the summer of 1941, Perrin H. Long, chairman of the National Academy of Science, Committee on Chemotherapeutic and Other Agents, wrote to his counterparts in Britain, asking them for information about recent penicillin research. His own committee was seriously considering investigations of the wonder drug. Leonard Colebrook wrote to Long from England (July 18, 1941): "I am shamefully in your debt for a report about chemotherapeutic drugs over here. I can only plead that there has been all too little to tell you, and I have been dashedly busy." Colebrook could only refer to what he called the work on "S"—the sulfanilamides—and said nothing about penicillin.

The British had more pressing concerns at the time. The Germans were threatening an invasion of Britain. Beginning in the summer of 1940, the German *Luftwaffe* pummeled Britain from the air, concentrating the attack on major industrial regions. Manufacturing capabilities of Great Britain were reduced to a fraction of their prewar levels. The summer of 1941 was no time for the British to begin a major penicillin industry. They lacked the time, ready capital, and personnel required for such a venture.

However, when the British mounted their counteroffensives in the wastes of North Africa in 1940 and 1941, the need for modern antibiotics was raised to the level of a national emergency. Florey had to look elsewhere for the sine qua non of all research—money. Research money was a constant worry for Florey. In the period from his first grant from the Medical Research Council, in 1927, to the late 1930s, when Florey sought funds for his penicillin research, he had been granted a total of £7,000 (Bickel, p. 237). When he applied in September 1939 for a grant of £100 to support part of the penicillin research, Florey was given to understand that he would receive no more than £25. He had also been turned down by the Nuffield Foundation and the William Dunn Foundation. The policymakers in the British foundations did not consider penicillin a viable project.

After the war, the penicillin program became a cause célèbre in Great Britain: several British scientists were castigated for having sold out British penicillin interests to the Americans. This is probably not the case. Florey went to the Rockefeller Foundation with the permission of Sir Edward Mellanby and Sir Henry Dale, both of the Medical Research Council. Both men realized that Britain would not be in a position to spend money on such speculative ventures as penicillin and hoped that the United States would be more likely to have the necessary money. In any event, John Wynden, writing for the London *Evening News,* expressed the popular dismay at Florey's awkward position: "Research in this country must be shamefully starved if an Oxford professor, for a paltry sum of less than £500 for sensational research work, has to go to the United States with a request for aid. . . . Our allies have a perfect moral right to exploit the discovery which only their financial support made a practicable affair" (Bickel, p. 237).

Florey had written to Warren Weaver at the Rockefeller

Foundation in the halcyon days of early 1936, requesting money for laboratory equipment. The work by Florey and Chain on lysozyme was just getting under way; the Rockefeller Foundation awarded them $1,280 in May 1936. When Florey's research group turned to the isolation of penicillin, the need for equipment became acute. In 1939, recognizing the potential uses of penicillin in the event of war, the Rockefeller Foundation awarded another $5,000 to Florey for further studies. This money supported Florey's first laboratory and clinical trials of the drug. With the likelihood of the United States becoming embroiled in the conflict, the need for antibiotics would become an international emergency.

On the strength of Florey's preliminary findings of the low toxicity and high therapeutic value of penicillin, the Rockefeller Foundation awarded Florey another $5,000 to finance his trip to the United States. At the time Florey proposed this audacious program, the amount of penicillin to treat a single person for one day required 125 gallons of fermentation broth. Without major innovations in methods for producing the drug, penicillin would remain a laboratory curiosity.

Florey brought Heatley, his microbiologist. Chain was not invited to go; in fact, Chain did not learn of the trip until Florey and Heatley were on their way.

Florey and Heatley could not have come to the United States at a better time. The feeling among scientists, administrators, and government officials was that a new age of science was about to dawn. Prior to World War II, basic science was a peripheral concern in the United States. Applied science and technology enjoyed the generous support of government and industry. Herbert Hoover estimated, for instance, that in 1930 the United States spent about $200 million a year on applied science and only about $10 million on research. Of the 35,000 scientists and engineers working at that time, no more than about 4,000 were involved in research and teaching (Greenberg, 1967, p. 52). By the close of World War II, however, American scientists had developed the conviction—and rightly so—that they had made an indispensable contribution to the war effort. Senator Claude Pepper of Florida, a champion of the role of big organized science in the national welfare, told Congress in 1945 that "it took a war of catastrophic dimensions to jar enough money out of the national pocket to enable medical research men to conduct their work on an adequate scale." Florey and Heatley arrived just as that pocket was beginning to open.

The era of the Yankee engineer, the gadgeteer, the tinkerer was ended by the relationship of government and science fostered by the exigencies of war—the atomic bomb, the MIT Radiation Laboratory, the National Advisory Council for Aeronautics, the Science Advisory Board, and the National Research Council—but all this was just getting under way when Florey and Heatley landed in New York. They were welcomed by a group of people who dimly recognized that they were about to seize the opportunity they had been waiting for.

The first stop on Florey's itinerary was the Rockefeller Foundation, where he conferred with his supporters and sought their help in collecting a group of U.S. scientists and manufacturers who might be interested in penicillin. The search took Florey and Heatley on a circuitous tour of the United States. From New York, Florey went to New Haven to visit with his children, who had been staying with John Fulton, professor of neurophysiology at Yale Medical School, in order to avoid the dangers of the war in Britain. Fulton introduced Florey and Heatley to Ross Harrison, president of the National Academy of Sciences. Harrison sent them to meet Charles Thom at the Department of Agriculture. Thom, finally, made the critical connection. He sent Florey and Heatley to meet with Percy Wells of the U.S. Bureau of Agricultural Chemistry and Engineering, who then sent them to the Northern Regional Research Laboratory of the U.S. Department of Agriculture, in Peoria, Illinois.

This relatively obscure government laboratory proved to be one of the most important contributors to the program to develop the natural penicillins. It had been set up during the Depression, at a cost of more than $2 million, to find commercial uses for agricultural products. In the words of a contemporary observer, "this object includes more than umbrella handles from milk. The laboratories are a development created by the Depression, an attempt to deal with surplus crops other than by burning" (J. H. Burn, *Newsletter* No. 35, August 7, 1943). Several factors recommended the laboratories at Peoria: they were becoming expert in techniques of deep fermentation, and they were interested in relationships between ingredients in the nutrient medium and the characteristics of the natural products grown in the fermentation broth.

Florey and Heatley arrived in Peoria on July 14, 1941. They met with Robert Coghill, head of the fermentation division, and in a short time decided that Peoria was indeed the place for their work to begin. Florey had his continuing responsibilities at Oxford and left for Britain in mid-September. Heatley stayed in Peoria. Research there went in two directions: finding a suitable medium on which to grow the *Penicillium* and adapting methods of deep fermentation, which were traditional in such industrial processes as beer brewing, to the special requirements of the *Penicillium* mold.

Florey had more or less adopted Fleming's original method for growing the *Penicillium* mold. He mixed the nutrient medium and seeded it with *Penicillium*. Within a few days, the surface of the medium would be covered by a dense mat of blue-green mold. Because 500 square centimeters of surface area were required for every liter of fermentation broth, the fermentation chambers used for growing *Penicillium* had to be specially built shallow vessels.

At one point, in desperation, the Oxford team used bed-pans, and the fermentation vessels designed for the job had roughly that shape.

Surface area was one of the principal limiting factors in the development of large-scale methods for the production of penicillin. Penicillin investigators also lacked a method for making *Penicillium* grow quickly. Either they had the wrong strain of *Penicillium* or they were using the wrong nutrients. Whatever the true source of the problem, the *Penicillium* mold grew slowly and required vast numbers of shallow fermentation dishes. And, to make matters worse, the penicillin finally produced was impure.

Heatley and Andrew J. Moyer, a staff scientist at the Northern Regional Research Laboratory, worked together on the problem of what to feed *Penicillium*. Their collaboration, however, was hampered by friction. In fact, after the close of the penicillin program, Moyer filed in his own name a British patent (Number 13674-6) for additions to corn steep liquor that were worked out with Heatley. Despite their differences, in a matter of weeks the two men made a startling discovery. "It is to be noted," they wrote in their collaborative report circulated late in 1941, "that this cooperative study has resulted in a greatly improved method for penicillin production whereby yields are increased twelvefold over those previously reported" (CMR general file). The key to their success was the discovery of a nutrient medium that favored the production of penicillin and was both plentiful and cheap.

The essential ingredient in the Heatley-Moyer nutrient medium was corn steep liquor, a by-product of the corn starch manufacturing process. Corn steep liquor is the liquid left behind after the corn is soaked and the corn kernel is removed. Moyer and Heatley found that this surplus by-product, mixed with neutralizing agents to keep the solution from becoming too acid as the penicillin grew, was just what the mold needed for rapid growth. Moreover, it favored the production of the effective penicillin G rather than the relatively less effective penicillin F and others. The recipe was simple:

| | |
|---|---:|
| Commercial glucose | 11.0–44.0 g. |
| Sodium nitrate ($NaNO_3$) | 3.0 g. |
| Magnesium sulfate ($MgSO_4 \cdot 7H_2O$) | 0.25 g. |
| Potassium dihydrogen phosphate ($KH_2PO_4$) | 0.50 g. |
| Concentrated corn steep liquor | 60.0 ml. |

$H_2O$ sufficient to make 1,000 milliliters of solution

The discovery that corn steep liquor was an excellent nutrient for *Penicillium* converted what had been a glut on the market, sold at the time for four cents a pound by the Corn Products Refining Company of Peoria, to a vital life-saving drug. The price of corn steep liquor, however, would soon reflect its importance. By March 1942, Heatley wrote to Florey in England that "the price of the stuff is 28 cents per pound. . . . I had the impression that it was a lot cheaper than that" (Heatley to Florey, March 21, 1942, OSRD CMR general file). Of greater significance than the price was the simple fact that the nutrient was working. Florey wrote back to Heatley from England that he, too, was having great success with corn steep liquor.

For years, corn steep liquor was treated as an essential wartime product; official price controls were not removed until October 1946. Two factors affected the decision to deregulate the substance: first, the war was over; and second, the magic ingredient in corn steep liquor had been discovered. Phenylacetic acid, present in corn steep liquor, could be furnished more cheaply by purely chemical means. The initial discovery by Northern Regional Research Laboratories, however, was probably the most important of several crucial discoveries made through the years of the penicillin program.

## Enter the Pharmaceutical Industry

When Florey and Heatley began their mission in the United States, the three leading pharmaceutical companies in this country were already considering involvement in the penicillin business. Merck, Squibb, and Pfizer had already begun experimenting with shallow culture methods in a desultory way. When Moyer and Heatley discovered how easily *Penicillium* could be prompted to increase the production of penicillin, the "Big Three" were quick to recognize the significance of the discovery.

On September 5, 1941, Richards began to act on the resolution by the CMR to investigate the possibilities of a large-scale research program to develop penicillin. The first step in such a program was to find out what interest could be drummed up in the field. To this end, Richards and the CMR organized a conference, officially called Microbial Therapeutics. Representatives of the Big Three and other pharmaceutical concerns attended: McDaniels, Stokes, Folkers, Peck, Woodruff, Robinson, and Benson. Florey and Heatley were guests of honor and primary sources of information at this historic meeting.

According to notes taken at the meeting by R. L. Peck, the following points were discussed:

1. Strains of *Penicillium* under investigation at that time had been carefully compared and consensus was that the *Penicillium notatum* discovered by Fleming remained the best of the lot because it was the easiest to grow and reliably yielded the most potent penicillin product.

2. The Peoria group had managed to increase the production of penicillin twelvefold after only six weeks of collaboration with Heatley. This improvement augured well for the future production of penicillin.

3. The pH of the broth in which the *Penicillium* grew profoundly affected the product. Penicillin is produced only if the concentration of hydrogen ions (pH) in the fermentation broth remains within a rather narrow range of values.

More subtle effects of pH were discovered. When Florey and Heatley visited the Merck laboratories in September 1941, for instance, Merck investigators told them that they were regularly producing penicillin at pH 3–4. The British investigators had been consistently finding penicillin production only within pH 5–7.5. In addition to this discrepancy in results, the Merck penicillin was white, not the green mold familiar to British scientists. "Dr. Florey expressed some doubt that the Merck product is really penicillin" (memo from A. J. Benson to R. T. Major, September 5, 1941, OSRD CMR general file).

Florey's upsetting news threw the American effort into confusion. "I am intensely interested in your opinion that the stuff that Merck's people have been working with is not the same as penicillin. If that is true, I hope with all my heart that they can be straightened out before long" (Richards to Florey, September 9, 1941, OSRD CMR general file).

A report issued considerably later by the Merck laboratories (OSRD general file) and bearing the epigraph from Kipling, "Anything green that grew out of the mould/Was an excellent herb to our fathers of Old," unraveled part of the mystery. A second antibacterial substance, called notatin, is produced when the pH drops below "a certain critical level and remains there." Other factors were introduced to further complicate the picture; considerable chemical evidence showed that British and American investigators were working with two different penicillins. Others would be discovered in time.

4. Purification of penicillin was still a problem, but progress was being made in describing the chemistry of penicillin. As the penicillin investigators were to learn in the coming years of research, they were mistakenly certain, at the time of their meeting, that the penicillin molecule contained only carbon, hydrogen, and oxygen. As far as the scientists attending the first meeting were concerned, penicillin was a middle-size molecule and not beyond the scope of the

chemist's art. "It was suggested," Peck wrote in his notes of the meeting, "that synthesis was probable but might require some rather long time—hard to say definitely, of course."

5. An appropriate method by which to assay the potency of penicillin was still lacking. Objective measurements of the biological activity of penicillin were impossible, and comparisons of various penicillins produced by different methods in different laboratories were therefore extremely difficult.

6. The mechanism by which penicillin worked to kill bacteria was still a complete mystery.

7. Application of the antibiotic in therapy was considered likely, although a great deal of clinical work would be necessary to determine toxicity and other potential hazards posed by the drug as well as proper indications for penicillin treatment, minimal effective dosage, and means of administering the drug.

### Cooperation

In the two months following the initial meeting, Richards organized several other meetings with whomever might be interested in penicillin *and* capable of making a contribution. Charles Thom, the leading authority on *Penicillium*, and representatives of Pfizer, Lederle, Merck, and Squibb attended the first such meeting on October 9, 1941. "It was agreed that the scientists connected with the four commercial companies were to report the deliberations of the conference to their respective companies and obtain a statement of their respective positions toward a concerted program of research on penicillin involving the pooling of information and results" (CMR minutes, October 9, 1941).

Informal and formal discussions that followed failed to resolve the thorny issues of coordinated research among several highly competitive pharmaceutical companies involved in a common research and development program. Richards held another high-level conference on December 17, 1941, at the University Club in New York with representatives of Squibb, Pfizer, and Lederle. "Understanding was reached that the organizations there represented should inform me from time to time of their progress in the production of a supply of penicillin" is all that Richards could report of that meeting (CMR general file). "Little was accomplished," Richards wrote, in organizing "a cooperative effort to produce enough of the substance for further clinical tests and for further chemical investigation" (letter to G. H. A. Clowes, December 22, 1941, CMR general file). (Richards sent the same message to Bush, Thom, and William Clark of the National Research Council.)

The strongest agreement that Richards and the industry could forge was described by Richards:

Careful consideration was given to the question of cooperative work with pooling of information and results. It was decided that if the companies retained independence of activity, the work would go forward as expeditiously as was necessary and that many troublesome questions concerned with commercial interests would be avoided. . . . It was agreed that each company should keep the CMR, through its chairman, informed in detail of the progress; that if discovery of such critical importance were made by any one company as to lead the Committee to the belief that the national interest required its disclosure to the others, the question of its disclosure would be taken up as an individual matter [December 22, 1941, Dir. Spec. Subj. Corres. file].

The operative clause in this agreement was "the belief that the national interest required its disclosure." That clause made the CMR arbiter in the delicate issue of disclosure of scientific information and in the protection of proprietary rights.

Richards had great difficulty in bringing the industrial interests together to cooperate on the joint production of penicillin. The flurry of patent applications concerning penicillin that appeared immediately after the war suggests that the companies involved were not completely forthright in their disclosure of penicillin research. They kept some of their best secrets hidden from public view. The distribution of raw penicillin for research and development was another problem. The major producers of penicillin saw some of their product going to competitors for research that might lead to better methods of penicillin production or even to synthesis. In other words, the major penicillin producers found themselves in the awkward position of fostering research that could very well injure their own commercial interests.

Strains also appeared between the public and private sectors of the research program. Investigators in the public domain came to resent the freedom with which the profit-making private sector could reap the benefits of their research. When the military and industrial situation required strict censorship of penicillin research information, the academic and government scientists further resented the limitations imposed on their publications.

Coghill wrote (to Chester Keefer, October 17, 1942) that "the boys here at Peoria" are working on the penicillin problem "on the seven-day-week basis" and complained that the exchange of information between the Northern Regional Research Laboratory and the Big Three was not satisfactory. "As far as we are concerned here at Peoria, it has been largely a case of giving all our information and receiving very little." Coghill further spoke out against the exclusivity of the Big Three. For example, Richards had instructed Coghill not to release to other laboratories studying penicillin any subcultures of the highly successful Squibb Strain No. 832, one that proved to be "decidedly superior in submerged culture work." Coghill replied that he suspected "a Squibb-Merck closed corporation [and] I feel very strongly that other people should have the benefit of this superior variant."

Almost a year later the problem of sharing information

continued to rankle. Richards wrote to another investigator at Peoria, H. T. Herrick, sympathizing with their predicament, but Richards also felt the need to remind his colleagues at Peoria that their installation is "a Governmental institution. . . and our services can therefore be expected to be made freely available. The commercial companies, on the other hand, . . . are private institutions not under contract to the Government and not in receipt of Government funds. They are wholly willing to share their information with the Government. We, however, under present conditions, do not have the right to distribute that information without specific permission." Richards closed his letter to Herrick on a more optimistic note: "I am hoping that a broader exchange of their information will shortly be made possible" (August 12, 1943, CMR general file).

The "broader exchange" remained a problem. As late as 1944, Richards asked Vannevar Bush to use his influence to ease the tensions developing between the group at Peoria and chemists in the pharmaceutical industry. By this late date in the penicillin program, the government scientists were objecting to the double jeopardy of neither enjoying financial reward that might accompany their important penicillin research nor getting their rightful scientific due. Richards wrote,

I have known for some time past that the workers under Dr. Coghill in the Peoria Laboratory who have done so much in laying the scientific foundations of the penicillin production program are uneasy and discontented because of restrictions on publication for which I have been largely responsible. . . . You are aware that it was to Peoria that Drs. Florey and Heatley went when they reached this country in 1941 and Florey made public acknowledgment of the help which Coghill's group has given. . . . The Peoria group has been the fountainhead of information to which producers turned for help in the beginnings of their operations. I know of no single group which is more worthy of recognition from the higher levels [June 10, 1944, CMR general file].

The issue never was resolved. Geography, history, and convenience conspired against the research group at Peoria. Merck dominated the research, and in general the Big Three influenced the course of the penicillin program.

By the end of 1941, nevertheless, with the entry of the United States into the war, the CMR was encouraged to believe that a penicillin program could be assembled. Richards asked the management of the leading commercial laboratories for their recommendations of who should be involved in the program. "No one can come in simply because he wants to," Richards said to Bush (memo of telephone conversation, December 17, 1941, CMR general file). "He has got to have a contribution to offer. We would be the judge of whether his contribution is enough to let him in. This means, in addition to a capacity to produce the stuff, he must have an admission ticket. When we think that enough companies have come in to do the job, we can stop."

What the "admission ticket" might be was no secret. At the time Heatley joined the scientists at Merck, late in 1941, George Merck assured Richards that the company was ready to spend $100,000 in equipment for penicillin production if the CMR asked him to (Richards to A. Baird Hastings, Department of Biological Chemistry, Harvard University, November 15, 1941, CMR general file). The Big Three—Merck, Pfizer, and Squibb—as well as Commercial Solvents, Cutter, Lilly, and Wyeth were ready to pay such an admission ticket. Other firms followed shortly as penicillin production became a national priority.

### Patents

National interest, military security, and proprietary rights became more confused as the penicillin program progressed. The natural penicillins were the domain of the independent commercial firms; the research in possible synthetic penicillins, on the other hand, was strictly controlled by the CMR. By 1944, progress toward synthesizing penicillin had been sufficiently encouraging to prompt Keefer to contact Dr. Frank B. Jewett, president of the National Academy of Sciences, to meet with the CMR and advise Bush on the question of patents arising from penicillin synthesis. This meeting took place on June 15, 1944.

Even though penicillin had not been synthesized by the end of the war, the proprietary battle was shaping up over the synthetic product. Interest in patenting aspects of the fermentation process for natural penicillin waned when, as production of natural penicillin multiplied and a surplus was created, the prices of penicillin came down. There were severe price wars as penicillin companies realized that they would be forced to either cut back on their production and shut down some production lines or keep the normal lines going but dump the surplus penicillin on the bulk market. This penicillin eventually showed up as competitive formulations by a host of new packagers and distributors. Penicillin G had no patent protection (Penicillin V was later protected) and was therefore available for any firm that might want to package and sell it.

Plans were formulated to use solid wastes of penicillin fermentation as a cattle feed, as a binder for blacktop, or as insulation. Bristol Laboratories actually looked into the possibility of industrial uses of penicillin. Penicillin could be used as a chemical resolving agent in the production of optically active organic materials. Unfortunately, the cost of penicillin was not quite low enough for that application, nor was penicillin durable enough for such purposes. It also was suggested that penicillin be broken down to penicillamine because penicillamine was found to be a good sequestering agent and even then was being used in electrolyte baths and other commercial applications.

Semisynthetic penicillins, on the other hand, were quite a different story. If important semisynthetic penicillins could be manufactured, the producer would want full patent protection of the process and, if possible, protection of the formula of the new penicillin itself. Consequently, as synthetic penicillins became likely—and, incidentally, as the war came to a close—the issue of patents became increasingly important.

In the international arena the guarantee of patent rights is not always simple. Toward the end of the war, therefore, British and American diplomats and lawyers worked feverishly to hammer out a document that would define the rights and obligations of all parties involved in the international penicillin research and development program. "I was glad indeed to hear that the 'legalities' have at last been pushed aside," Sir Henry Dale wrote to Richards in August 1944, "and that the accumulated information about Penicillin chemistry has been passing both ways. If these war necessities can only establish a whole-hearted scientific cooperation between our countries, that will be a positive gain of tremendous value, to set against so much that is being wrecked for generations" (August 2, 1944, CMR general file).

Agreements had to be written between the United States and Great Britain, partners in the cooperative venture to develop the natural penicillins and to come up with a commercially feasible means of synthesizing at least one of them. In a letter to the Under Secretary of State E. R. Stettinius, Jr., Bush once again called attention to the need for "steps to be taken to insure a fair disposition of patent rights and the full protection of our [American and British] mutual interests. We propose, accordingly, to continue our negotiations with representatives of the British Government with a view both to formalizing our present agreement and to working out the details of the many patent problems resulting from the interchange of information between us" (draft, CMR, July 27, 1944). Further agreements were necessary between the United States and the Lend-Lease countries, who stood as direct beneficiaries of American aid in the postwar reconstruction.

At the close of the war, penicillin was an open secret. Suddenly plants were being built all over the world: Portugal, the Temple of Heaven in Peiping, Argentina, Bombay, Brazil, Spain, India, Chile, and many other places. By 1946, the British were exporting an estimated 370 million units of penicillin a month to what remained of the British Empire and to continental Europe (*New York Times*, July 10, 1946). That same year, exports from the United States amounted to an estimated $10 million.

Almost as soon as penicillin came out from under strict government control, a thriving black market in the drug developed. The first recorded attempt to export penicillin without a license—that is, smuggle—was detected in the end of March 1945. Treasury customs agents seized 26 million units of penicillin at Laredo, Texas, waiting to be shipped illegally out of the country (*New York Times*, March 31, 1945). On a smaller scale, Julio Henriques Futuro, a Portuguese seaman, was arrested for allegedly smuggling 200 vials of penicillin out of Philadelphia (*New York Times*, June 24, 1945). A seaman working out of New York was accused of trying to sell 300 vials of penicillin on the Cuban black market. He would have made $25,000 (*New York Times*, June 5, 1946).

The most elaborate penicillin racket was run in Berlin just after the close of the war. American and British intelligence agents discovered a ring of thirty-two Germans involved in selling counterfeit penicillin. A bottle of crushed atabrine (an antimalarial drug) in a penicillin bottle sold for about $800. A bottle of glucose sold for $1,000–1,500 (*New York Times*, April 21, 1946, and May 6, 1946).

By 1948, however, the price of penicillin had fallen so low that the bottom fell out of the black market operation. The German operation had involved millions of dollars; later black market deals involved only thousands.

# 4 The Impossible Problem

Without the intervention of scientific reasoning in the development of drugs, pharmacology could never have been formulated along rational lines. As in present-day folk medicine, the pharmacopeia would be a compendium of knowledge about natural products that had worked in the past, but such knowledge would not permit the prediction of classes of chemical compounds that might work in the future to alleviate pain and combat disease.

The discovery of the sulfa drugs represented a significant advance in medical science because sulfa research allowed chemists to identify a molecule capable of killing bacteria in the body without injuring every other cell within its reach as well. The development of the sulfa drugs were important, too, because, after having identified such a discriminating molecule, chemists could run seemingly endless changes on the basic molecular theme, altering properties of the substance to suit particular medical needs. The idea of synthesizing penicillin was more audacious than that of synthesizing the sulfa drugs, and the possibilities presented by penicillin were even more impressive, given the special properties of that molecule. The sulfa drugs were wholly the product of chemistry; penicillin was the creation of living organisms. In attempting the synthesis of penicillin, chemists were forced to reproduce one of life's complex products. Not long ago, people firmly believed that, as the famous nineteenth-century chemist Berzelius said, "an impassable gulf" separated the living from the inorganic worlds. So profound was this belief that for a long time the definition of organic chemistry depended on it. Not until the latter part of the nineteenth century did the term *organic* refer simply to compounds manufactured by living systems or more generally, to the chemistry of carbon compounds.

One would have thought that by the time the penicillin problem presented itself, chemists would have long since abandoned their archaic vitalist assumptions. But the amazing success of the natural fermentation program and the endless frustrations encountered in the chemical synthesis of penicillin led serious scientists to doubt whether a penicillin synthesis was even possible. Chronic frustration does odd things to people. In the case of the penicillin synthesis program, it revived the early belief that nothing but the tissues of living organisms could form the substances extracted from living creatures and that no process invented by human art could imitate the compositions found in organic mysteries of plants and animals.

The penicillin molecule, at first apparently so simple, proved to be beyond the reach of art. As late as 1946, Ernst Chain told a meeting of British scientists that he could not imagine an artificial alternative to the natural penicillins. Synthesis of penicillin, he said, would probably not be possible because "the 4-membered ring that contains the marvelous biological properties has resisted concentrated efforts of the hundreds of chemists now working on it." Synthesis of the penicillin molecule, he went on to say, must unfortunately remain beyond the reach of chemistry "unless someone invents an entirely new technique now unknown to chemistry" (*New York Times,* July 5, 1946, vol. 17, p. 8).

Three years before Chain uttered these pessimistic remarks, the future of penicillin synthesis did not seem so bleak. "One of the greatest scientific prizes in modern times awaits those who will achieve these goals [of synthesizing penicillin]; for the finding of the chemical pattern of penicillin may give the clue to a host of other chemically related substances that may make the sulfa drugs very crude by comparison" (William Laurence, *New York Times*, August 1, 1943, IV, p. 5). Thus "the greatest scientific race is going on among the laboratories," wrote Laurence, to determine the chemical structure of penicillin, "a step necessary before any substance can be made synthetically."

### The Next Necessary Step
In October 1943, the OSRD, working through the CMR and in collaboration with the British Medical Research Council, agreed to mount "a coordinated attack on penicillin synthesis." This program, of course, was a direct extension of work already in progess on the natural fermentation of penicillin. The synthesis program, like the fermentation program, was to be protected by strict secrecy for military and proprietary reasons; consequently, little was known about it during the war years. The OSRD research on the synthesis of penicillin was purely what we would call today mission-oriented research. When the success of the naturally fermented penicillins and the success of the military campaigns were both assured, the government-sponsored program to study the chemistry of penicillin and to synthesize the compound was no longer appropriate. The OSRD penicillin synthesis program was terminated on November 1, 1945. After the war, the success of the natural penicillins eclipsed progress made on synthetic penicillin, so the story of the massive government program to synthesize the drug has been known primarily to the participants.

Despite the apparent failure of the penicillin synthesis program, it remains a fascinating chapter in the history of American science. Scientists and government agencies cooperated closely for years, doggedly determined to solve a problem that became more difficult the more scientists worked on it.

Why would the Big Three of the pharmaceutical industry—Merck, Pfizer, and Squibb—attempt the expensive venture of synthesizing penicillin when they had already spent very large sums of money in working out the highly successful methods for natural fermentation?

I think that the history of the industrial production of the B vitamins may give the answer. In the 1930s the Merck group built a plant to produce vitamin $B_1$ (thiamine) from rice hulls. Of course, there was a serious medical demand for vitamins, and the pharmaceutical houses went to work to satisfy that demand. But even in areas where beriberi and other vitamin deficiencies were not likely to present a real medical problem, vitamins had become popular supplements to the diet, guaranteed to ward off everything from cancer to the common cold. The Merck plant, however, never went into production for the purpose of manufacturing vitamin $B_1$ from rice hulls because that installation could not compete with the newly developed synthetic process. By the early 1940s, not only the B vitamins but vitamin C and other natural products were synthesized industrially. Synthesis proved far more reliable and cheaper than isolating compounds from natural sources. At great expense Merck converted their plant to some other purpose, and the management was mindful not to repeat the mistake.

When chemists learned that penicillin was not a large molecule and, in some ways not a very complicated one, the total synthesis of penicillin became commercially attractive. For the Big Three, in other words, work on the total synthesis of penicillin was simply a defensive move to protect their own positions. They would assure themselves, by carrying on vigorous research programs on the chemistry of penicillin, that if anyone were to synthesize the penicillins and thereby undercut the commercial hegemony enjoyed by the fermentation product, it would be one of the Big Three. By formally and informally cooperating in the basic research, moreover, the Big Three might all enjoy success if they were to unravel the mysteries of the penicillin molecule.

Merck and Company was the acknowledged leader in the

research effort. George Merck was not a chemist, but he was a good businessman. He knew how to attract talent. One of his most talented managers was Randolph T. Major, hired in the 1930s as director of research. He had great vision and a genuine feel for what were going to be important problems in the immediate future. He had very good judgment of the abilities of the people around him to carry out scientific projects. And when necessary, he could attract the best consultants available to supplement the expertise of his own already impressive group. Both Vannevar Bush and A. N. Richards, for instance, were consultants at Merck, at one time or another.

Major's particular slant in managing the pharmaceutical research at Merck was to strengthen the relationship between the disciplines of biology and chemistry. He was responsible for gathering a group of men and women who shared this particular view: Max Tishler, Karl Folkers, Jackson Foster, Boyd Woodruff, Jeff Webb, Joseph Stevens, and a number of other capable scientists. Major's research team prospered so that by the end of the 1930s Merck and Company was unquestionably the finest research laboratory in the pharmaceutical industry. Research conducted there rivaled, and in some ways probably surpassed, research programs in the best academic laboratories in the country. Merck was probably the only pharmaceutical company seriously dedicated to pure and applied research on a large scale. Many of their competitors were still formulators, pill rollers, and had not come up with a major pharmaceutical development in their entire history. It was no surprise, then, that Merck would assume the lead in penicillin research. The penicillin problem was made to order for the Merck research philosophy and personnel.

In 1943 the great advances in natural production of penicillin had not yet reached their fullest potential. Production was faster, yields were greater, and the price of penicillin was coming down, but authorities on both sides of the Atlantic were haunted by the fear that penicillin production would not keep pace with military and civilian demands. In the words of one popular writer at the time, "The only hope of easing this situation lies in synthesis. If chemists can make the drug artificially, large supplies would be immediately available" (Ratcliffe, 1943). If the active chemical responsible for the magic of penicillin could be isolated and then synthesized in the laboratory, as the *New York Times* editorial stated (September 3, 1943), "we could dispense with the mold-growing entirely. That is the next step."

Alexander Fleming himself recognized this next logical step and urged chemists to work toward synthesis of penicillin. Speaking to Americans in a transatlantic radio broadcast (December 14, 1943, on the occasion of his receiving the Award of Distinction from the American Pharmaceutical Manufacturers Association, presented by Major Norman T. Kirk), Fleming proclaimed that the future of penicillin lay in the chemists' laboratories. "The chemists will fasten on the molecule and modify it, as they have done with the sulfanilamide molecule in the last five years, so that derivatives of penicillin will appear more powerful, or with wider applications, and diseases now untouched will be conquered" (*New York Times*, December 14, 1943, vol. 13, p. 1). Likewise, Florey, addressing the Royal Society of Arts a year later, said that a practicable synthesis of penicillin was the only means by which to satisfy the growing military and civilian demand for the drug. "Progress in making the substance synthetically is being made," he said, "but nothing more can be said now, since it is on the secret list" (*New York Times*, June 8, 1944, p. 4).

Military secrecy was only one reason that so little could be said. Progress on the chemistry of penicillin had not been as rapid as the chemists or the administrators might have hoped. The penicillin molecule proved to be a formidable puzzle.

## The Penicillin Synthesis Program

From the earliest days of the penicillin program, the scientific and pharmaceutical community recognized that the *Penicillium* mold was capricious, slow growing, and difficult to domesticate. Moreover, the penicillin it produced was diluted manyfold by the fermentation broth so that the antibiotic was found in extremely low concentrations and was difficult to extract. Several methods were available for concentrating small amounts of penicillin in the laboratory, but the problem of extracting the large quantities that would be necessary in industrial production, was not easily solved.

One solution to the extraction problem was a device known as the Podbielniak extractor. This is a rather tall column, basically a large counter-current column, in which two immiscible liquids are passed against each other. By means of an elaborate system of baffles and inlets and outlets, the extractor separates penicillin from the impurities in the broth. Once it was recognized that several different types of penicillin were produced at the same time, the Podbielniak extractor was used to separate the various penicillins from each other. The Podbielniak extractor was used in a few pilot plants but was much too cumbersome to work with once simpler chemical methods of extraction were discovered.

The Podbielniak devices would have remained a footnote in the chemical history of penicillin had it not been for the Cold War battle fought over them. After the war, Poland, Czechoslovakia, and Yugoslavia complained to the United Nations World Health Organization (*New York Times*, March 3, 1949) that policies of the United States prevented their buying this essential piece of penicillin production equipment. The United States position was "Security considerations are involved. We have no further comment at this time" (Francis E. McIntyre, Assistant Director, Office of International Trade, *New York Times*, March 3, 1949). Uruguay, the Philippines, and Norway complained as well. But despite a unanimous vote by the World Health Organization deploring the U.S. action (*New York Times*, April 27, 1950), the United States remained adamant. The Podbielniak extractors would not be exported.

During the 1940s, the principal research effort was directed toward preparing the purest penicillin salt possible. My research group at Merck, which included W. J. Mader and Donald Cram, developed a process using the so-called metathesis reaction between an N-ethylpiperidine salt of penicillin G and a solution of sodium or potassium 2-ethylhexanoate. The rearrangement of radicals on these two molecules produced the sodium or potassium salt of penicillin G in highly purified form. Before we discovered this method, however, Dr. Oskar Wintersteiner's group at Squibb had succeeded in crystallizing penicillin G. Squibb therefore had a corner on the market, selling what they maintained was pure penicillin G. Our own experiments, however, showed that their product was only 85 percent penicillin G, the remainder was a mixture of other penicillins and contaminants carried over from the fermentation broth. When our own purification process was used, Merck was able to produce a penicillin G that was almost 100 percent pure.

Although we had come a long way in isolating and purifying the penicillins, most scientists working with penicillin would have preferred working with a purely synthetic product, which could be tailored to our needs, would be relatively easy to handle, and could be produced in almost endless supply. In 1943 the consensus was that if the history of penicillin were at all like that of the vitamins, a synthetic product would eventually be far less expensive to produce than the naturally fermented product.

By August 1943, Vannevar Bush found himself at what he called an "impasse" because chemically pure natural penicillin could finally be prepared, and yet the synthetic penicillin held the brighter promise. "Experimental results continue to be startling," Bush wrote (August 21, 1943, Dir. Spec. Subj.

Corres. file). "The stuff has now been crystallized." Two years earlier, Karl Meyer had showed Robert Coghill what Meyer alleged to be crystals of penicillin. Coghill, however, said that even with the aid of a high-powered microscope, "I was not convinced of the crystalline nature of his preparation" (Coghill to Richards, December 27, 1941, CMR general file). The product looked more like a powder than like crystals. Coghill could see no sharp edges, points, or clearly delineated faces. But the more recent experimental findings coming from Oskar Wintersteiner's laboratory were incontrovertible. Penicillin G had finally been crystallized.

In August of 1943, Richards sent the following memorandum to his committee:

Synthesis. Crystallization accomplished by Squibb. Indications point to possibility of earlier accomplishment of synthesis than thought possible a few months ago. May have it in a year. 15 kilos of pure substance would equal 30,000 million units [August 14, 1943, Dir. Spec. Subj. Corres. file].

A few months earlier Coghill had written to Richards that the penicillin molecule was apparently not as large as was formerly thought, "which is encouraging from the point of view of synthesis. The way things look at the moment, . . . I am gradually coming to the conclusion that penicillin will eventually be synthesized rather than produced by fermentation. This, however, is merely an opinion" (Coghill to Richards, April 12, 1943). Coming from the man whose laboratory had contributed so much to the success of the fermentation program, however, this was a powerful opinion.

With the synthesis of penicillin within relatively easy reach—or so Bush thought in those heady days of late 1943—success itself posed serious problems. Hence Bush's "impasse." The immediate problem would be that of assuring an adequate supply of penicillin during the awkward interval while industrial plants tooled up for the chemical synthesis of penicillin. "The commercial companies," Bush wrote (August 21, 1943, Dir. Spec. Subj. Corres.), "would naturally be reluctant to spend a lot of money for plants that may be obsolete, yet the needs of the Armed Forces, to say nothing of civilian needs, demand that the stuff be produced at once and in quantity." There was also the problem of re-tooling those penicillin plants already in operation. Richards asked Bush, "How can compensation be arranged for the scrapping of present plants?" (memorandum from Richards to Bush, August 14, 1943, Dir. Spec. Subj. Corres. file). The answer is not recorded.

And the pooling of information? According to Richards, Merck and Squibb were already collaborating with each other. Pfizer was involved on a more limited scale. "Otherwise there is no pooling" (memorandum from Richards to Bush, August 14, 1943). The Big Three, at any rate, were already deeply involved in a more or less cooperative effort to study the chemistry of penicillin, with a view toward eventually selling the synthetic product.

Bush's strategy for controlling the situation was to give the CMR full authority over the penicillin synthesis program, just as all research projects and reports concerning penicillin were being passed through the CMR. Raw materials required for studies of penicillin chemistry also had to be requested from the CMR. Because Merck was to continue as one of the major sites of penicillin research, especially chemical investigations, Richards directed the U.S. Bureau of Priorities, Division of Industry, War Production Board (WPB) in February 1942 to give "the highest possible priority" to Merck's penicillin projects so that "eventually it can be made in chemical laboratories" (Richards to C. H. Matthiessen, Jr., Chief of Bureau of Priorities, WPB, February 28, 1942, Dir. Spec. Subj. Corres. file). Although other firms were brought into the penicillin program, Merck continued to enjoy this privileged status.

Roger Adams was chosen to direct the penicillin synthesis program. He was an excellent choice in the view of most people involved in the project. One critical voice, however, argued that Adams had never "been up against the problem of working on the structure and synthesis of a naturally occurring material of which only a tiny amount of the pure crystalline substance is available" (Robert E. Waterman to Carroll L. Wilson, OSRD, September 22, 1943, Dir. Spec. Subj. Corres.). The criticism was unfounded. Working independently of Alexander Todd, Adams had elucidated the structure of delta-9-tetrahydrocannabinol (except for the location of one double bond) in 1940. He also studied gossypol, a poisonous substance found in cotton seeds. Probably the most important factor in choosing Adams, however, was that he was one of the most knowledgeable and influential organic chemists of that generation. He had a large research group at the University of Illinois, from which many students went to become influential chemists in their own right. At one time, it seemed that DuPont was dominated by Adams's protégés. Adams had also founded and edited since the years of World War I two indispensable annual volumes, *Organic Syntheses* and *Organic Reactions*. Reactions appearing in those two publications had the weight of canon. Many chemists referred to Adams as the Pope of chemistry and his board of editors as the College of Cardinals. Robert D. Coghill and Hans Clarke shared with Adams the responsibility of directing the CMR synthesis program.

As in the early days of the penicillin fermentation program, finding the necessary expertise, facilities, and interest throughout the pharmaceutical industry was the first order of business. Hans Clarke and Roger Adams were therefore sent by the CMR to the likely pharmaceutical houses in late 1943 to survey the situation and to determine which groups could be expected to make most rapid progress in the synthesis of penicillin.

Clarke and Adams visited Merck in October. In their report to Richards (October 12, 1943), they said that they were "both much impressed" by what they had found at Merck. They found that Randolph T. Major, director of research, was eager to continue penicillin work, especially since the emphasis had been shifted from natural fermentation to chemical synthesis. Karl Folkers, head of the Fundamental Research Group at Merck, had at least four highly trained and imaginative investigators under his direction. Bob Peck and his three assistants would work on the extraction and isolation of penicillin. Don Wolf and his assistant would do the necessary microorganic studies of the structure of the penicillin product. Ralph Mozingo and his two assistants would be in charge of the degradative and synthetic studies. Jeff Webb and Nelson Trenner were already at work on the constitution and physicochemistry of penicillin. In short, Clarke and Adams found that penicillin was a lively issue at Merck when they made their visit. "Speculations with regard to the structure were unreservedly propounded and discussed," they reported.

Clarke and Adams went to Squibb as well. The Squibb laboratories, they said, did not seem so well "organized" as those at Merck, but Clarke and Adams were nevertheless impressed by the talent they found. George A. Harrop, director of research, put his research staff at the disposal of Clarke and Adams. Oskar Wintersteiner, head of the Organic Chemical Division, could supply a competent staff. H. B. MacPhillamy, who had done the actual laboratory work to crystallize the sodium salt of penicillin, would continue his chemical studies of penicillin. J. D. Dutcher would be the microorganic chemist of the group. H. E. Stavely, who had been primarily interested in sterol chemistry at the time, would begin working on penillic acid. Marjorie Anchel would be in charge of the synthetic studies.

By November 1943, Merck, Squibb, and investigators at Oxford University had isolated important parts of the penicillin molecule so that "a few reasonably plausible structures can now be formulated." The CMR Penicillin Committee expected a decision within a few weeks, but "certain unusual features in its chemical behavior may possibly give rise to unforeseen difficulties which could be re-solved only by synthetic methods. We therefore believe that more of the outstanding chemical talent in the country should be available to the problem" (report of the CMR Penicillin Committee, November 6, 1943).

At roughly the same time, an unidentified member of the CMR (perhaps Richards) wrote the following unsigned, un-dated memorandum of a conversation. The document can be found among the CMR papers at the U.S. National Archives.

1. Is penicillin degradation and synthesis a war-time prob-lem? Yes—Synthetic production, if accomplished, cannot be expected sooner than two years. War may well be over in two years. But: Discovery of constitution may point to other compounds, accessible during the war which may have po-tency similar to that of penicillin. . . .
Question: Are university chemists needed?
Answer: Yes.
Question: Why?
Answer: 1) Some have unique experience and ability. 2) Public opinion may well demand that such an important matter be not left wholly to company chemists.

The memorandum concludes:

5. Can problem be divided into A) Degradation and B) Synthesis, and free exchange be limited to A? Doubtful.
6. Choose one laboratory (e.g., du Vigneaud's) as working center. Enlist Carter, Bachmann, Doisy as consultants. Choose Squibb and Merck and Pfizer as nucleus of com-panies [OSRD CMR general file, late 1943].

The CMR did precisely what was outlined in the memorandum. Their criteria for selecting laboratories for the nucleus of the program was that they be large enough to assure a sufficient number of organic chemists but not so large that security would become a problem. According to CMR documents, they had three reasons for wanting only moderate-size laboratories: larger numbers of people working on the project might "endanger the security of secret information"; large laboratories might "embarrass the control" of patent information ceded to the OSRD; and an unmanageably large operation might lead to wasteful duplication of effort.

Ten companies were enlisted in the synthesis program: Abbott, American Cyanamid, Lilly, Merck, Parke-Davis, Pfizer, Roche, Squibb, Upjohn, and Winthrop. Four academic chemists were recruited as general consultants: W. E. Bachmann (University of Michigan), H. E. Carter (University of Illinois), R. D. Coghill (Northern Regional Research Laboratory), and V. du Vigneaud (Cornell Medical School). Bush wrote to Richards only three months after his "impasse" to say that "I feel that the penicillin situation is now in good shape" (December 4, 1943, Dir. Spec. Subj. Corres. file).

Less than two years later, the penicillin program was terminated. In late summer 1945, the contractors working on penicillin received letters from Bush saying that "Current military developments have changed the status of the penicillin-synthesis program." Contracts would be terminated. There would be "no further formal demand" for the penicillin information, which had been submitted to the CMR as a matter of routine, except for the mandatory final research report. Patent provisions, however, would remain operative, although the rest of the agreement could be considered nullified. Bush commended the chemists for their "patriotic unselfishness and international goodwill which has characterized our collaborative effort" (August 27, 1945, OSRD CMR general file), and with that brought to a close one of the most remarkable research programs in the history of science.

### The Chemistry of Penicillin
The development of penicillin follows in general the historical path of organic chemistry from natural substance to

synthetic product. The early dyes mauve and indigo were probably the first natural products to be studied extensively by chemists; magenta and a number of other dyes were studied soon afterward. In each case, the work of the chemists was an attempt to free the users of the product from depending on rather unpredictable natural sources. By improving the basic material, both in purity and chemical structure, chemists could devise better dyes than nature herself had constructed.

Chemists have often found themselves in the role of first attempting to duplicate the natural product and then improving it. For instance, the development of an artificial silk had been a long-time goal of chemists. The synthetic rayons, although having many of the desirable qualities of silk, were at first inferior to silk in strength and durability. In recent years, some rayons have been so improved that they are fully competitive with silk. The next step in the development of artificial fibers, however, was to emancipate chemists from the natural product entirely. Instead of trying to imitate silk, as they had done with rayon, chemists created an entirely new substance, with desirable properties of its own— namely, nylon.

One of the conceits of mankind is that nature has created its diverse products for human use. Silk is a good example. The silk worm obviously creates the silk for its own purposes. Couturiers exploit the work of the silk worm for use as a textile fiber, but this was not the silk worm's intention. The concept carries over to the field of medicine as well. Although alkaloids and other substances have been isolated from plants to cure malaria (quinine), relieve pain (morphine), or to combat human infection in human beings (antibiotics), they are part of the physiology of the plant, not part of our own. Considerable effort is thus involved in appropriating the products of such organisms to our own uses.

The goals of the penicillin synthesis program were the classic goals of organic chemistry. The first goal was to identify the compound. Fleming made the first step in this direction. Once he had subcultured enough penicillin, he began a study of its chemistry. In his first scientific communication on the subject of penicillin, he reported that the penicillin he isolated was soluble in water and alcohol but not in ether or chloroform. From this and other chemical evidence we can now infer that Fleming was working with the salt form of penicillin and not with the free acid. He also observed that penicillin was most stable when in a neutral solution, acid and base would disrupt the molecule and destroy the antibiotic properties.

During the following decade, little new information was added to the meager store of knowledge about the chemistry of penicillin. Percival W. Clutterbuck, Reginald Lovell, and Harold Raistrick found that penicillin could be extracted with ether if the acidity of the solution was carefully controlled. They also found that oxidants and other factors would readily deactivate penicillin so that all of the antibiotic properties were destroyed. Furthermore, they found that penicillin could be adsorbed on charcoal.

This was the sum of knowledge about the chemistry of penicillin when Abraham and Chain began their work on chemical aspects of the penicillin problem in early 1940. It had been shown by this time that penicillin could be re-extracted from an organic solvent into water at a neutral pH. This had been shown by Dr. L. B. Holt in Fleming's laboratory in 1934. The Oxford team did not know of Holt's work at the time, and Heatley independently re-invented the Holt extraction process. Nobody had yet succeeded in isolating and purifying penicillin; nor, of course, did anyone have the slightest idea of what might be its active principle.

Robinson, Abraham, Baker, and Chain devoted themselves to the elucidation of the chemical structure of the penicillins and to the synthesis of some of their degradation products. The methods of classical chemistry in the 1940s were cumbersome, perhaps, but they served well. When chemists working with penicillin found themselves baffled by the molecule, the problem was not with the methods. Rather, we suffered from a peculiar blind spot, a chemical prejudice that prevented our appreciating the true value of the data we had before our eyes. On several occasions, we went on ignoring the facts because we could not believe that the structure of penicillin was what the data indicated.

The first challenge for chemists was to determine the size and molecular weight of the penicillin molecule. Several different laboratories found that penicillin was a relatively small molecule with a molecular weight of no more than 300–400. A molecule as small as penicillin, we thought, could be readily described and, as we somewhat innocently believed, could be synthesized without too much difficulty.

The next step was to determine what atoms and how many of each comprised the penicillin molecule. Penicillin would certainly contain carbon and hydrogen and was likely to contain other atoms as well. After performing what they considered to be exhaustive qualitative and quantitative tests, Abraham, Baker, Chain, and Florey hazarded the opinion in 1942 that the formula for the barium salt of penicillin was $C_{24}H_{32}O_{10}N_2Ba$. At just about the same time, chemists at Merck proposed a similar formula. Almost immediately, however, chemists at both Merck and Oxford withdrew their formulas because they realized that impurities in the original material rendered the chemical tests meaningless.

The main source of difficulty was that until we learned how to handle the penicillin molecule, the more we treated it, the more we lost. As a result, we were careful to do as little to the penicillin as possible. Successive precipitations in hopes of getting a relatively pure penicillin unfortunately led to degradation and rearrangement of the starting material.

A discovery made in 1942 in several laboratories emphasized the importance of nitrogen in the chemistry of penicillin. The biological activity of penicillin was directly proportional to the nitrogen content of the sample. This was an important clue; but what it might mean was not at all obvious to chemists trying to puzzle out the structure of penicillin.

Abraham and Chain, in the meantime, refined their analytic techniques and came up with another formula for penicillin: $C_{23}H_{20}O_9N_2$. In the United States, Karl Meyer, working at Columbia, had completed his series of analyses of penicillin and suggested a pair of possible formulas: $C_{14}H_{19}O_6N$ or $C_{19}H_{17}O_3N$. Meyer described penicillin to Coghill as "a very unstable polyhydroxyaromatic acid of molecular weight approximately 500, containing more than one nitrogen, but no sulfur or phosphorus."

With this tentative information, chemists tried valiantly to arrange the atoms into a plausible structure. Nothing worked. Either there was too much latitude in assembling the pieces, so that no unique solution to the problem presented itself, or there was too little freedom and the pieces would not fit. The parts of the penicillin molecule seemed to be falling into an apparently impossible structure. More information was needed before we could give a reasonable description of the penicillin molecule.

One of the standard methods of determining the structure of a complex molecule is to subject it to harsh treatment and then study results of the destruction. By analyzing fragments of the penicillin molecule, we hoped to fit the fragments together, as one would assemble a jigsaw puzzle, to yield to structure of the original. Chemists in the United States and in Great Britain dissolved the penicillin salt, in the purest form they could obtain at the time, in strong acid and boiled it for approximately an hour. Three degradation products were identified: carbon dioxide, the salt of a base, and a volatile acid. The base was given the name penicillamine, because it was quickly apparent that that fragment was an amino acid (and hence the portion of the molecule containing the nitrogen). J. H. Burn described this experiment in his secret report to the OSRD (*Newsletter* No. 2, January 31, 1943). "Chain and Florey have recently described the isolation of a breakdown product, a nitrogenous base having properties related to ascorbic acid. It reduces similarly to ascorbic acid. It gives a characteristic blue color with ferric chloride which is not given by many other substances. Certain hydroxyaldehydes give it and reductive acid also gives it. The substance contains half the nitrogen in the molecule, and is called Penicillamine; it is a kind of amino sugar, and it has been crystallized. Its molecular weight is about 250 and its formula is something like $C_6H_{11}O_4H \cdot HCl$."

The discovery of penicillamine was an unexpected boon. In one easy step, the chemists had characterized what appeared to be about half the penicillin molecule.

The second big surprise came soon after chemists on both sides of the Atlantic redoubled their efforts to describe the chemistry of penicillin. Joseph F. Alicino at Squibb dried penicillin, burned it, and analyzed the ash. He found, as expected, a complicated mixture of cyanide, carbonate, and so forth. He then added sulfuric acid to sulfate the ash and performed the normal Pregl analysis of penicillin, in which the penicillin is oxidized in a closed system with oxygen flowing over the sample. To his amazement he found that the sulfated ash weighed the same as the initial untreated ash. That experimental finding could only mean that sulfur was already present in the penicillin molecule. When chemists oxidized penicillamine with bromine, a compound known as penicillaminic acid was formed. When this compound was analyzed, all the formulas for penicillin were proved wrong.

With a shock of recognition, chemists found that the penicillin molecule contained sulfur as well as carbon, hydrogen, oxygen, and nitrogen. "We have recently isolated a beautifully crystalline, sulfur-containing organic derivative of a large part of the penicillin molecule," Frank Stodola of the Peoria laboratory wrote to Richards (August 17, 1943). "It was inconceivable to us that the Oxford and Merck investigators would have neglected to test their degradation products for sulfur."

"Chain and I missed the presence of sulfur in 1942," according to Dr. Abraham, "because the microanalysts in the Dyson Perrins Laboratory reported that our best preparation of penicillin was sulfur free. At our first meeting with Sir Robert [Robinson], he asked us if sulfur was present and we told him of the report of the analysts. In retrospect, of course, we should not have accepted the analytical report so readily. The presence of sulfur was established in Oxford in July 1943. We were not aware of American work at that time" (personal communication).

The failure to recognize the presence of sulfur in penicillin was a classic blunder. When the discovery was verified, many faces were red. I think that one of the problems must have been the impurity of the product with which they were working. No analysis of penicillin could be definite until a pure crystalline product could be prepared. Penicillamine, on the other hand, was readily crystallized and yielded the definitive proof that sulfur was present in that important portion of the penicillin molecule.

The question remains for some chemical sleuth, how did the best chemists of the time miss the presence of sulfur in penicillin? I have a guess, but it will require some laboratory work to prove. If they were using the barium salt of penicillin in the elementary analysis, it is just possible that barium sulfate could be formed, and barium sulfate would not give the characteristic precipitate of lead sulfide when treated with lead acetate.

Ironically, Clutterbuck had reported the presence of sulfur in his 1932 report on the chemistry of penicillin (Percival W. Clutterbuck, Reginald Lovell, and Harold Raistrick, CCXXVII. "Studies in the biochemistry of microorganisms. XXVI. The formation from glucose by members of the Penicillium chrysogenum series of a pigment, an alkali-soluble protein and penicillin—the antibacterial substance of Fleming," *Biochemistry Journal,* 1932, vol. 26, pp. 1907–1918). Clutterbuck had isolated a "crude nitrogenous substance," which he purified, dried, and analyzed. The substance was composed of carbon, at 51.51, 51.76 percent; hydrogen, at 6.85, 6.95 percent; nitrogen, at 12.75, 12.95 percent; and sulfur, at 1.35, 1.32 percent.

Knowing that penicillin contained an atom of sulfur (atomic weight 32) meant that all previous formulas for penicillin contained two atoms of oxygen (atomic weight 16) too many. Knowing that the penicillamine portion of the penicillin molecule contained the sulfur, moreover, located the important sulfur at the business end of the penicillin molecule.

The discovery, shortly after, that penicillamine was invariant, regardless of what type of penicillin it came from, reinforced the notion that penicillamine was an essential part of the penicillin molecule. Side chains might give the various penicillins their distinctive properties, but the heart of the matter that made penicillin the antibiotic that it was had something to do with the penicillamine. This was a sufficiently promising lead, and in 1943 it prompted the OSRD to begin formally its penicillin chemistry and synthesis program.

Once we had found that sulfur and nitrogen coexist in the same major portion of the penicillin molecule, penicillamine, we asked what compounds do we know that contain sulfur and nitrogen? The quick answer was the class of compounds known as thiazolidines.

Thiazolidines had been in the chemical literature, at least as a scientific curiosity, even since the German chemist A. Hantzsch discovered the five-membered rings in 1887. They had not attracted great interest, however, until Clarke and Ratner re-investigated them in the 1930s. By another of the coincidences that determined the history of penicillin, Clarke, the man who was to direct much of the chemical research on penicillin, had studied, purely by chance, one of the major constituents of that molecule years earlier. Even when Clarke and Ratner carried out their research, the thiazolidine ring was considered an obscure structure.

Thiazoles, the more highly unsaturated, pseudo-aromatic ring systems related to the thiazolidines, had a somewhat more glamorous role in chemistry. Workers in the dye industry, especially in Germany, had studied thiazoles empirically over the years. Dye chemists had been searching for an efficient chromophore, the color-bearing portion of the dye molecule, and consequently investigated a wide assortment of ring systems. There was considerable interest in aromatic groups because they made it easier for dyes to attach themselves to molecules of the fabric to be dyed. Hence, the interest in thiazoles. When the thiazole ring structure finally showed up in nature, in the 1930s when the structure of vitamin $B_1$ (thiamine) was worked out, interest in thiazoles and related structures began to grow.

Elementary chemical analysis showed that degradation of penicillin yielded the thiazolidine penicilloic acid.

Desacylpenicilloic acid.

Familiar chemical reactions could be adduced to relate penicillamine to the newly discovered product, penicilloic acid. A major piece of the puzzle had fallen into place.

Penicillamine.

Other degradation products of penicillin were being identified and studied. The most important ones were penicilloic acid, as we have seen, and the so-called penillic acids. More pieces could be fit into the puzzle. Since penicillamine was known to be about half the penicillin molecule, we were sanguine about the possibility of discovering the complete structure of the molecule in a relatively short time.

The chemical and physical behavior of penicillin was

Known degradation products of penicillin.

studied and furnished important information about the possible structure of penicillin. We found, for example, that penicillin had a single acidic function (the carboxyl group, $-COOH$). Degradation products, on the other hand, were found to be dibasic. Those findings could only mean that the penicillin molecule had a bound form of the carboxyl group, but in a form that was easily liberated. We also knew that the carboxyl group in the penicillin molecule was in the penicillamine portion. Finally we found that the atoms of the penicillin molecule would readily rearrange to form a ring containing two nitrogen atoms.

One of the most incredible aspects of the penicillin story is that discovering its molecular structure turned out to be so difficult. Very early in the research program the major degradation and rearrangement products of penicillin were identified and isolated: penicillamine, penilloaldehyde, penicilloic acid, penillic acid, phenylacetic acid, and carbon dioxide. Several other products of chemical reactions with penicillin were also identified. Most of these products had also been synthesized. Nevertheless, despite the fact that there seemed to be so few pieces to the penicillin puzzle, and despite the fact that we were already familiar with the degradation and rearrangement reactions involved, we could not agree on a probable structure for the penicillin molecule.

The leading contender by the end of 1942 was the combination of two rings proposed by Abraham, Chain, Baker, Robinson, and others at Oxford, the oxazolone-thiazolidine. At almost the same time, chemists at Merck proposed the identical structure. Given the presuppositions and prejudices of chemists at the time, the oxazolone-thiazolidine was the most likely structure. The proposed structure contained the familiar five-membered thiazolidine and five-membered oxazolone. As Chain was to say in his Nobel Lecture in 1946, the proposed structure was not only reasonable in itself but it depended upon a "plausible reaction mechanism

Oxazolone portion

Thiazolidine portion

Oxazolone-thiazolidine formula.

for the penillic acid rearrangement suggested by Sir Robert Robinson." But there was a serious problem with the proposed structure: the oxazolone-thiazolidine formula predicted that there would be at least one basic group in the penicillin molecule. No such group could be found by potentiometric titration. As the "plausible" rearrangement reaction seemed less and less likely, the penicillin molecule began to take on less than familiar properties.

A second possible structure for penicillin was suggested by chemists at Oxford and Merck. This slightly different assembly of rings known as a beta-lactam-thiazolidine structure accounted for the chemistry of penicillin better than did the oxazolone-thiazolidine, but it was a wholly unfamiliar beast. Beta-lactams had never been found in nature, and no familiar chemical reactions could explain how the observed degradation products of penicillin could be fit back together again to yield a beta-lactam structure. Nevertheless, as the potentiometric titrations devised and run by Jeff Webb and Nelson Trenner at Merck showed, something was dreadfully wrong with the oxazolone-thiazolidine formula.

The simplest beta-lactam then known, 2-azetidinone, showed absolutely no biological activity. This fact blinded us.

Beta-lactam formula.

Even when we tried the desperate measure of using a Grignard reagent (a class of organomagnesium halides, which are highly reactive compounds) to cyclize beta-alanine, I think many of us were secretly relieved to see that the beta-lactam formed in the reaction showed no promise of getting us closer to a synthesis of penicillin. The possibility was too outlandish.

Because both pieces of what was believed to be the penicillin molecule—the familiar oxazolone ring and the equally familiar thiazolidine—were known. And since the sequence of so many of the atoms of penicillin had been established by degradation and synthesis, we believed that their linkage would be fairly obvious.

I had been doing some work on that type of structure when I was at Merck. What other people not so familiar with the idiosyncracies of the oxazolone structure had failed to recognize was that no known oxazolones had a substituent arranged as the sulfur group would be in the penicillin molecule. Such molecules seemed to rearrange spontaneously to form an unsaturated oxazolone.

In addition to the virtue of familiarity, the oxazolone-thiazolidine formula had a powerful champion, Sir Robert Robinson. On first acquaintance, Sir Robert gave the impression of an English gentleman. Karl Folkers has characterized him well.

I was very fond of him as a person. I went to Oxford two or three times to see him, and it always was a great personal delight. He had taken us into the Mitre Hotel, that old hotel in Oxford, for what we would call a cocktail. He was not supposed to be drinking anything alcoholic. But he wanted something, just sherry, so he left his wife someplace else and took my wife and me into the Mitre.

I remember going into that laboratory of his in Dyson Perrins, through some laboratories where he had a private laboratory. The room had a strange shape. It was not rectangular or square, it was something unusual. So we went into the office, and with the greatest of ease he started drawing structures and talking reactions for a long period of time until he had had enough. Incidentally, his guest had had enough too.

One time when it came time to go down to the railroad station, I had a fairly heavy bag with me. Sir Robert grabbed my bag to take it out to his car. I could scarcely bear the thought of this famous man carrying my suitcase. It was my job to carry that suitcase. But there was no way I could convince Sir Robert of that. He grabbed it and he insisted upon carrying it. He was not so young, even at that time. I felt I should carry my own bag. But no, here was this great man, carrying my very heavy bag out to the car.

Sir Robert was formal and even courtly; but if he were crossed in any way, and especially in a discussion of chemistry, his personality transformed instantly. At such times, Sir Robert was an opponent to be reckoned with. By anyone's judgment, Sir Robert was a brilliant man. This comes through in his earlier work on such molecules as morphine, plant coloring materials, and some of his pioneering suggestions on what is now known as physical organic chemistry. In addition, he was a first-class chess player. He carried out chess matches with a number of prominent players throughout the world by mail and, on occasion, would play several simultaneous games. Even the most brilliant people have their blindspots, however. Sir Robert simply refused to allow the possibility of any penicillin structure but the oxazolone-thiazolidine.

Despite chemists' familiarity with oxazolone-thiazolidine, neither formula could capture the field. In February 1944, Coghill wrote to Clarke, "We are very skeptical of the azlactone- [another term for oxazolone] thiazolidine structure and feel that there is a very unstable and biologically active molecule which rearranges under very mild inactivation conditions to the thiazolidine structure. We have no quarrel with the work which has been done, as it all seems to rest on a very solid foundation, but I think you will grant that there are reasons for believing that the active principle is not a thiazolidine" (February 17, 1944).

Not a thiazolidine! The one secure starting point for all the chemical work done to date on the structure of penicillin was called into question. Chemical compromises were proposed.

Frank Stodola, working at the Peoria laboratories, proposed a structure "something between an azlactone and a lactam," according to Coghill. Stodola and Coghill were appropriately tentative, however, in recommending it. "Please do not infer from this," Coghill cautioned Clarke (February 17, 1944), "that Dr. Stodola and I are sold on his proposed formula. We merely feel that, from the point of view of the degradation products, it has certain advantages over the other formulas, and should not be overlooked in the present unsettled state of affairs." W. E. Bachmann, working at the University of Michigan, saw considerable merit in Stodola's compromise. His was an ingenious attempt to resolve the dilemma. But the compromise, unfortunately, was not a penicillin. Coghill was ambivalent. In that same letter to Clarke he finished by writing, "I recently visited Steve Ballard and the Shell group at Emeryville [California]. They are certainly sold on the beta-lactam structure, and I must admit that they make it look pretty good." The Shell group had been studying the infrared spectra of Hermann Staudinger's beta-lactam compounds. They were probably leading experts in the physical determination of beta-lactams.

At this point, the CMR enlisted the help of R. B. Woodward, *wunderkind* of organic chemistry at the time. Woodward suggested that a careful study of the heats of combustion—a measure of the potential energy contained in the chemical bonds—of the oxazolone ring might allow chemists to at least rule out that structure. Clarke solicited the help of Frederic Rossini of the U.S. Bureau of Standards.

Tricyclic formula.

"I remember Woodward and that tricyclic formula with some amusement," Folkers has said, "because his fame was somewhat substantial, even then. Everybody rushed to synthesize something like that formula instantly. There was an immediate turnaround. Many, many laboratories in America and in England took over the tricyclic formula, simply because Woodward put it forward." However, the tricyclic formula was only one possibility by Woodward, who clearly favored the beta-lactam structure.

### Wandering among Rings

By 1945 there was a good deal of indirect evidence to support the beta-lactam structure, but direct evidence was still lacking.

When the synthetic penicillin programs were in full swing,

the British would regularly send a delegation to meet with their American counterparts. I remember one meeting at Merck. At one point, Sir Robert Robinson was at the blackboard. He had the floor and was giving his arguments in favor of the oxazolone-thiazolidine structure of penicillin. I suppose because I was still young and brash, but also because I had been doing some work on the oxazolone-thiazolidine structure in connection with a possible synthesis of penicillamine, I said, "Sir Robert, the oxazolone-thiazolidine is not only not the correct formula for penicillin, it is an impossible structure. It will never be synthesized, at least not in the sense that you will be able to put the product in a bottle and store it at room temperature." Sir Robert was taken aback at hearing this from such a small shot. He brushed me aside, as he often did, with counterarguments and managed to put me in my place.

Two methods of obtaining direct evidence of a chemical structure were available at the time. The first was the traditional method of organic chemistry, that is, to synthesize the compound according to a rationally derived formula. In the case of penicillin, the formula that could be synthesized would obviously be the correct formula. A second method for deciding between the two structures, still new in the 1940s, was X-ray crystallography.

Toward the end of 1944, the OSRD arranged for a small supply of penicillin to be sent to Dorothy Crowfoot Hodgkin, of the Department of Mineralogy, University Museum, Oxford. She would undertake a single-crystal X-ray study of the structure of penicillin, which would require months of single-minded application and might still result in an uncertain outcome. Her X-ray study would involve sending a beam of X-rays through a single crystal of a salt of penicillin. X-rays passing through the molecule would be bent by constituents of the molecule and form diffraction patterns, which she would record photographically. By arranging the photographic records of the patterns in a way that made chemical and physical sense, Dorothy Hodgkin could furnish positive evidence for the structure of penicillin. Today the computer can do the busy work, manipulating the diffraction patterns. In the 1940s, this manipulation had to be done by cutting photographs of the figures and moving them around on a table until a satisfactory pattern was recognized.

Despite the time, money, and precious penicillin the project would require, Coghill and others at the OSRD were willing to take the chance. Moreover, the beauty of the X-ray technique was that it would furnish a positive picture of what the penicillin molecule looked like. If Hodgkin found anything at all, her findings would be conclusive. On December 18, 1944, a sample of "NRRL 12-18-44," penicillin X, was shipped to Dorothy Hodgkin.

The OSRD, however, brought the penicillin program to a close before she finished her research. W. H. Kennerson, executive secretary of the Committee on Chemotherapeutic and Other Agents, wrote the discouraging memorandum (April 12, 1944) on the "importance of penicillin in the war effort." "Notwithstanding the intensive efforts to elucidate fully the chemical structure of penicillin," he wrote, "and to produce it by synthesis, the production of penicillin for the present and so far as we can see into the future, depends directly on the continued production of the microorganism *Penicillium notatum*."

Malaise spread throughout the industrial and academic laboratories. The government agencies, too, were beginning to apply their resources to other problems. Penicillin came to be known as the "impossible problem" and was put aside.

"The actual chemical work is at a low ebb among our groups," Carter wrote to Clarke from the University of Illinois (April 24, 1945), "although the biological precursor work is being pushed rather vigorously. I don't know what the sentiment is elsewhere, but I would say that most of our men feel that the synthesis of penicillin is now a long-range proposition on which it is difficult to maintain any great enthusiasm. Most of the men are suffering a reaction from the high-pressure efforts which they made during the last year or so. This has certainly been a strikingly unusual problem in every way. I suppose it is only fitting that that should be so in view of the unique biological properties of the molecule. I only hope that we will crack the problem some day."

### Triumph of the Beta-Lactam

Three approaches to elucidating the structure of penicillin did finally pay off: The definitive *chemical* experiment was the desulfurization performed by Mozingo; the definitive *physical* work was done by Dorothy Hodgkin; and the definitive *physical-chemical* experiment was the potentiometric titration carried out by Webb and Trenner, which revealed no basic properties. According to Karl Folkers, "it was Ralph Mozingo who really conceived the idea of removing the sulfur atoms from such organic compounds with Raney nickel. He used to talk about that sort of thing; but the organic chemists in the lab were not inclined to take it seriously. And so the months were ticking by without anything definitive in terms of structure. Finally, in those early days of doing all kinds of things to penicillin, and on the basis of Ralph's interest, penicillin was finally treated with Raney nickel. But the experiment was not successful."

We would find out later that there was a kind of competition between the opening of the beta-lactam ring by hydrolysis and the removal of the sulfur atom in a desulfurization reaction. In those early experiments, it was largely a matter of the penicillin molecule being hydrolyzed instead of losing its sulfur.

"In a period of chemical frustration, not knowing what to do next, we were sitting around the lab," according to Folkers, "probably some evening after doing the day's work."

I don't know who came up with the idea, but I'm sure Kaczka was there, Ralph was there, [Don] Wolf, [Stan] Harris, and myself. We were the key chemists there at the time. Somebody said, "Why don't we get everything ready with freshly prepared Raney nickel catalyst?" The idea was to get a preparation of Raney nickel catalyst that was as saturated with hydrogen as could be. Ralph said that he would make some. Then, instead of trying to run the desulfurization at a low temperature, which would allow the hydrolysis to become the main reaction, somebody said, "Let's heat that solution very quickly to a reflux temperature. Fast. And then, after a few minutes, let's cool it down fast in ice water. Get the temperature up fast, to accomplish the desulfurization, and then cool it down in a hurry to terminate any hydrolysis that might take place." We were pretty sure that the desulfurization would take place quickly.

Of course, we had our eye at that time on the beta-lactam formula, so we knew what to expect when we removed the sulfur. Harris and Don, between them, synthesized the desulfurization products for comparison with those obtained from the penicillin. It was all done over the weekend. By Monday, as far as I was concerned, it was all over. We knew that the beta-lactam was the right formula.

The triumph of the beta-lactam was not an easy victory; in fact, even after the definitive work had been done, investigators had trouble accepting it. The Shell infrared work was probably the first evidence that revealed the lactam carbonyl. That was clean research, but the significance of it was not appreciated at the time. Organic chemists were more convinced by the desulfurization.

Another piece of evidence for the beta-lactam came from the physicochemical research. A physical chemist at Merck, Jeff Webb, pointed out that of the many formulas that had been proposed for penicillin, only the beta-lactam did not have a basic group on it. Max Tishler thinks that Webb's observation was the significant one at the time; if only other investigators had recognized it. Even after the X-ray work done by Dorothy Hodgkin established, without question, that the beta-lactam was the correct formula there was controversy. As Karl Folkers said,

This all boils down to whether or not one accepts organic evidence as proof of structure. Under ordinary conditions this would be accepted, but the penicillin problem had proved so difficult, the ordinary evidence was considered insufficient. There was also a kind of intellectual, competitive interest between the X-ray and the organic determinations. If you were an X-ray crystallographer, you didn't accept the organic evidence; you accepted only your own data. If you were an organic chemist, then you would appreciate the significance of the removal of the sulfur atom from the thiazolidine.

Karl Folkers was convinced at an early date that the beta-lactam was the correct formula.

The first time I took the beta-lactam formula seriously was when I was on my way to visit Homer Adkins in the hospital. Homer Adkins had been a consultant to the Merck labs. I also took my graduate work with him. In all of my studies with him, Homer impressed upon me that there were only two kinds of chemistry, organic chemistry and physical chemistry. Biological activity was almost anathema to him.

In due time, Homer's personality, which captivated so many people, captivated Randolph Major, who was my boss. Major was always in favor of attracting good consultants. In those days, he had many of them. Homer found that our type of research was really very interesting. Something like penicillin, which was important because of its biological activity and its potential value in medicine, in due time captivated Homer, as it had captivated all of us.

About a year before Homer died, he was taking one of those penicilloic acids, dissolving the substance in some suitable medium, and subjecting the solution to ultrahigh pressure reactions in the Bridgeman style. He felt that maybe under such great pressures, he might get a somewhat higher yield of ring closure. About that time, he made one of his periodic visits to Rahway. We always exchanged laboratory results. I kidded him a bit. I said, "My goodness, Homer, you're running some new research here based on something that is biologically interesting. How come?" He replied with a laugh, "Well, I can learn too, can't I?" In the last year of his life, Homer became completely enthusiastic about organic chemistry that had biological overtones.

His diet was bad. He ate very badly; he consumed great

amounts of chocolates and God knows what else. Then finally he overtaxed his heart. So when I learned that he was in the hospital and was not expected to live, I went out to Chicago by train and then on to Madison. On the train from Chicago to Madison, I sat there, looking out the window, wondering what I would say to my professor. He knew that he was not going to live, and I knew. What, then, is there to talk about?

I could think of only one thing to talk about, and that was penicillin. So I thought, well, to go into the room and talk to him about the pros and cons of the structure of penicillin would be something that would interest him, and me, and would keep our minds off the health problem. As I reviewed the evidence in my mind about the beta-lactam formulas, they sounded pretty good. Of course, we had not yet done the desulfurization. So in his hospital room, we discussed the merits of the beta-lactam structure. We did this for no more than ten or fifteen minutes, and then I excused myself.

That was the last time I saw him. He died not long after that. It was on that trip that for the first time in my participation in the penicillin program, that I really took the beta-lactam seriously.

Chemical and physical evidence mounted in favor of the beta-lactam. The coup de grace was dealt the old oxazolone-thiazolidine formula by Dorothy Hodgkin's X-ray projections. Once she compiled all her pictures of the penicillin molecule there could be no further doubt. The beta-lactam had finally been demonstrated.

With the controversy of the structure resolved, however, a new controversy arose to take its place. Chemists on both sides of the Atlantic claimed to have been the first with the conclusive evidence. Abraham made claims for his work.

My memory is clear that having done the potentiometric titrations, and being unable to find any basic group, I wrote down the beta-lactam formula and went to Chain. That was in 1943. I said to Chain, "I think that this must be the structure." We had to admit by this time that there were only two reasonable structures: the beta-lactam or the oxazolone. So I said to Chain at the time, on the basis of the evidence coming from the titrations, that it must be a beta-lactam. Then we went to Wilson Baker in the Dyson-Perrins Laboratory and talked about writing our report. Both structures were mentioned in the report because although we were sure that the correct structure was the beta-lactam, we were also certain that Robinson wanted the other structure to be the right one. As a result, we wrote a rather neutral report. It would not have been fair to Robinson to have written the report with his name on it and not to contain the oxazolone because, after all, it was his structure. In fact, he wrote an appendix to the report disclaiming the beta-lactam structure.

In that famous PEN Report 103 (October 22, 23, 1943), the party in favor of the beta-lactam structure wrote a fairly weak case. After presenting evidence for the oxazolone-thiazolidine formula, they wrote, "Other formulae are possible and have been considered. An alternative formula for penicillin appears to explain in a natural manner its known properties. The easy formation of penillic acid from penicillin would involve opening of the strained 4-membered ring and ring closure to give (II) [a drawing of the beta-lactam structure appeared here]." The paper carries Robinson's addendum, "One of us considers the four-ring formula above somewhat improbable."

Dorothy Hodgkin supports Abraham's claim.

Right at the beginning Abraham and Chain thought that the structure was the beta-lactam. I had, of course, warned Sir Robert Robinson from time to time that it looked as if the data indicated the beta-lactam. But when that moment of complete certainty came, I went across to see him. He was still quite incredulous. He said, "You must have inactivated the material in the crystal. It must have changed in the crystal through the action of the X-rays." And I said, "Well, that is very easy to test. I will just take some of the crystals which we have exposed to the X-rays over to the laboratory and see whether they are active or not." It was quite interesting getting the test measured, because it made me think while I was waiting for the answer. If it had not been for this strong opposition, we would have been certain of the structure a long time before. It was just the weight of Sir Robert's opinion and the fact that his opinion influenced our approach. He not only influenced my approach, but that of Tommy

Thompson and Cornforth. But finally the answer came back from the laboratory, and the material was still active.

On the American side of the Atlantic, several chemists hold claim to first deducing the beta-lactam structure. The desulfurization work done by Mozingo gives him rightful claim to the honor. Jeff Webb's electrometric titrations, like those done by Abraham and Chain, give him a claim.

Throughout the debate Sir Robert believed that the stress on the beta-lactam would make the molecule impossible. I remember sitting across from him at a dinner for chemists in 1952. At the end of the dinner, just to make conversation I asked him if he had read my paper on a total synthesis of a 5-phenylpenicillin. He replied, "Yes, I read it. The paper was very interesting, but I have one small question. Why did you call it a penicillin?" "I called it a penicillin," I said, "because it has the complete penicillin structure. It simply has an extra phenyl group, but *penicillin* would certainly be the simplest way to describe it." At this, Sir Robert pulled himself up in his seat and said, "That compound cannot be a penicillin. It is a beta-lactam." I reminded Sir Robert that penicillin had already been shown to be a beta-lactam by chemical and physical methods. I also reminded him of the X-ray work done by Dorothy Hodgkin, to which he replied—and this is the brilliance of the man—"That is the result when the penicillin is in the solid form. You simply do not know what it is when the penicillin is in solution." I found it impossible to get the better of Sir Robert in any discussion of chemistry, even when I was right and he was wrong.

### A Synthetic Penicillin

Another of the ironies of penicillin history is that a synthesis based on the avowedly wrong formula for penicillin brought the penicillin synthesis program to a close. Merck reported to the world on January 31, 1944, and again, jointly with the Oxford group, on February 29, 1944, that synthetic oxazolones had demonstrable biological activity. Yields were extremely low: the best yields were in the range of 3 or 4 units per milligram, which compared unfavorably with the concentrations of penicillin produced naturally in the range of 1,500 to 2,000 units per milligram. Nevertheless this synthetic substance somewhat resembled a natural penicillin.

A few months earlier rumors of the synthesis spread through the community of chemists. There was excitement at the annual meetings of the American Chemical Society in Pittsburgh in September 1943, "when the rumor spread among the chemists that penicillin A [sic] has already been synthesized by a large pharmaceutical house. No confirmation could be obtained of the report which, if true, would be one of the greatest milestones in man's age-old struggle against disease. . . . If such a synthesis has actually been achieved, it was pointed out, it may very likely be kept a military secret for the time being" (*New York Times,* September 10, 1943, p. 6).

After years of struggling with the intractable penicillin, chemists came to believe that a synthesis was indeed possible. If the synthetic oxazolone had some small degree of biological activity, they reasoned, fusing the oxazolone with the thiazolidine must enhance the antibiotic properties and thus account for the dramatic difference in biological activity shown by the two compounds. The chemical problem, therefore, was simply that of joining the two rings, the oxazolone and the thiazolidine, to form what they mistakenly believed was the correct formula for penicillin.

With success apparently imminent, the CMR tightened the reins of its control. A discovery of such scientific and commercial importance, according to the CMR, could not be left entirely in the hands of the industrial interests. Academic chemists had already been brought into the penicillin program, and the CMR decided to allow Vincent du Vigneaud, at the Cornell Medical School, to take the public credit for fusing the oxazolone and thiazolidine rings.

In November 1946, du Vigneaud announced that he had produced a synthetic penicillin. The *New York Times* ran the story on the front page. "One of the greatest achievements in biochemistry," said the *Times,* for which du Vigneaud deserved full credit was that of duplicating in the laboratory the mysterious product of the *Penicillium* mold (November 8, 1946). *Newsweek* (1946, vol. 28, pp. 66–68) proclaimed that Fleming's "fabulous green mold" had been tamed. "No longer a delicate, frond-like substance, unsubstantial and elusive to the touch," penicillin was at long last an "artificially produced chemical that a scientist's fingers can reform, elaborate, and twist to his own ends."

Even amid the popular rejoicing, however, there was doubt and incredulity throughout the scientific community. Karl Folkers tells the story.

I got to know du Vigneaud prior to penicillin, when we were working on biotin. He and Klaus Hoffman, [Donald B.] Melville, and maybe one or two others were working on the isolation of biotin. They finally managed to retrieve a few milligrams of not very pure stuff. In the Merck laboratories, John Keretczky almost singlehandedly isolated beautiful stuff, absolutely fantastic. Not only that, but we could get something like fifty to a hundred milligrams every week, on the week, without fail.

Major, in his usual philosophical approach of cooperation, decided that we at Rahway should cooperate with du Vigneaud. So I went to Cornell and let it be known to D [du Vigneaud] that we had the stuff, a hundred milligrams every Friday. They had worked for months on end at Cornell to get smaller quantities of much less purity. We obviously had the ace in our hands.

That led to our working together on the proof of structure. D was not very keen on my working on the structure in Rahway and his working on it in New York. I had a structure man, whose name was Don Wolf, who would go into New York and work in du Vigneaud's lab. I talked with Don almost every day about what was going on in the lab and what we were going to do next. On Fridays, I went to New York and we had a Friday conference at D's place.

All of that work gave birth to the reaction of sulfur compounds with Raney nickel, thought up by Ralph Mozingo. We had used it in a definitive proof of the structure of biotin. The desulfurization proved the structure of biotin in a decisive way. The same chemistry was applied to penicillin. The only difference was that you could heat biotin with almost any medium and Raney nickel and there was no hydrolysis of the biotin. Penicillin was very, very readily hydrolyzed; and so we thought up the method of heat-it-up-fast and cool-it-down-fast to get the sulfur out of penicillin.

Du Vigneaud was not the first to assemble the two rings in an attempt to synthesize penicillin. Several chemists had already accomplished the same reaction; but for a variety of reasons, they all abandoned that route to synthetic penicillin. Karl Folkers and Stan Harris, in fact, hold a U.S. patent on the synthesis of penicillin along this route. "But," said Folkers, "it was probably the lowest possible yield an organic reaction ever gave. It remained for du Vigneaud, several years later, using the Craig counter-current distribution, to repeat that reaction on which we held the patent, to scale it up a bit, and with the counter-current methods to isolate the product and prove that it really was penicillin. That was always, I thought, one of the most amusing bits of chemistry in the whole penicillin affair."

The basic reaction that du Vigneaud and his co-workers used had been tried in four or five laboratories during the World War II effort. The Merck laboratory, Bachmann's laboratory, Sir Robert Robinson's laboratory at Oxford, and probably one or two others had tried the obvious route of putting the penicillamine portion of the molecule together with an oxazolone. Everyone who tried the reaction met with some success. The synthesis, however, was not a rational one; that is, it was not planned step by step using known reactions. It was a stab in the dark.

But by some strange sequence of reactions, not understood to this day, these components did indeed yield trace amounts of what was definitely shown to be benzyl penicillin (penicillin G). Two different approaches had been tried,

Oxazolone

Penicillamine

Oxazolone-Thiazolidine

Schematic summary of an early attempt at synthesis.

both motivated by the incorrect oxazolone-thiazolidine formula. In addition to the direct condensation, chemists attempted to remove the elements of water from penicilloic acid and its derivatives to close the ring. Both reactions produced minute quantities of penicillin G, perhaps because they pass through a common intermediate structure capable of rearranging, to a severely limited extent, to a penicillin. This common intermediate is most likely penicillenic acid, the reactions of which are probably the most extensively and intensively studied in the history of chemistry.

Rearrangement involving penicillenic acid.

In the closing months of the World War II project, and shortly after, word got around that du Vigneaud was re-investigating this reaction in spite of the fact that it had been so exhaustively studied in a number of laboratories. I knew of chemists who worked exclusively on that reaction for a year or more. They did nothing else but try every method that had been published, and some that had not been published, to bring about the condensation of the penicillamine and the oxazolone.

What was puzzling to those of us who had been involved in the earlier work was why anyone would re-investigate this reaction that seemed to be a thoroughly dead end. All the known methods had been tried by skilled chemists and had been found wanting. In spite of that, we found that the rumors of du Vigneaud's work were true. Du Vigneaud apparently repeated the condensation on a very large scale. We jokingly surmised that he must have been running the reaction in a bath tub. And that must have been roughly the scale. Then, taking advantage of the new counter-current extraction method worked out by Lyman C. Craig for isolating minute amounts of product, du Vigneaud was able to isolate about 14 milligrams of the benzylpenicillin. The triumph, I think, belongs to Craig for having developed the means of extracting such a small amount of product and not to the synthesis itself.

In a sense, du Vigneaud took credit from other laboratories. His publication—which, incidentally, he carefully called "Synthetic Penicillin" and not "The Synthesis of Penicillin"—based on the work of many different laboratories, received the full measure of attention from the popular press. Even the scientific press, kept in the dark about most of the developments in penicillin chemistry during the war, failed to acknowledge the work of other laboratories and gave the laurels to du Vigneaud exclusively.

The most important deficiency of the du Vigneaud reaction was that its mechanism was totally obscure. Although no one could doubt that the reaction had produced a trace of penicillin, no one could explain where the penicillin had come from. And the yield was a tiny 0.008 per cent. This small yield, in itself, is not a serious criticism of the reaction. The criticism was that not only was the initial yield low but, because no one knew the mechanism by which the reaction proceeded, no one could devise ways of improving the yield. Finally, the reaction failed as a rational synthesis of penicillin because the fundamental strategy was wrong: the premise of the reaction was that the oxazolone-thiazolidine was the correct structure of penicillin. Even as du Vigneaud was running his experiments, the final proof was coming in that the correct formula was a beta-lactam.

It is, of course, dangerous to judge du Vigneaud's motives in reinvestigating this reaction and then publishing the results with such ballyhoo. A few chemists felt that du Vigneaud's was a somewhat cynical operation: that he realized the experiment did not add anything to the picture because it had already been established that penicillin G was formed in small amounts. He did not attempt to increase the yield or to understand the mechanism of the reaction. Perhaps the reaction was run and publicized to give the CMR something to show for its massive investment in the program to synthesize penicillin.

An additional feature of the du Vigneaud episode in 1948 was that there had been a good deal of discussion and politicking among the scientists who had done their work during the World War II effort under secrecy required by the OSRD. These scientists had no opportunity to publish any of their scientific results under their own names. Everything was classified work and, although it eventually saw the light of day in the much abbreviated form appearing in *The Chemistry of Penicillin,* it was nevertheless not the same as having independent and full scientific publication of the research work. The publication by du Vigneaud broke the pattern. Apparently he was able to gather his own work together and publish it independently of the larger penicillin effort and under his own name. The work had to be cleared for publication, but Hans Clarke, standing at the gate, was reluctant to prevent scientists from publishing their findings. I do not believe that Clarke or any other member of the CMR was aware of the furor du Vigneaud's work would cause in the popular press. I am sure that they were taken by surprise, too, by the howls of anguish raised by the diligent scientists who had had their own penicillin work suppressed by the OSRD, once they saw du Vigneaud publishing his own work.

Nevertheless, justice prevails in the affairs of science. Even as the du Vigneaud achievement was being publicized, evidence was mounting to show that the oxazolone-thiazolidine structure was the wrong one. The beta-lactam structure was demonstrably superior to the other. Infrared absorption, thermochemical data, X-ray projections, and the desulfurization all proved that what was thought to be an impossible structure was nevertheless the correct one. The old oxazolone-thiazolidine formula was finally laid to rest. The chemistry of penicillin, and later the chemistry of related antibiotics, became the chemistry of the beta-lactams.

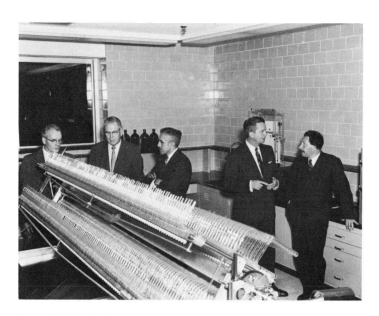

Inspecting the Craig counter-
current extraction apparatus at
Bristol Laboratories are (right to
left) Ernst Chain, John Sheehan,
and Amel Menotti (vice-president
and director of research at Bristol). The extraction method was
worked out by Lyman C. Craig,
and Vincent du Vigneaud used
the Craig counter-current distribution to obtain trace amounts
of penicillin in an attempt to prepare the oxazolone-thiazolidine
formula.

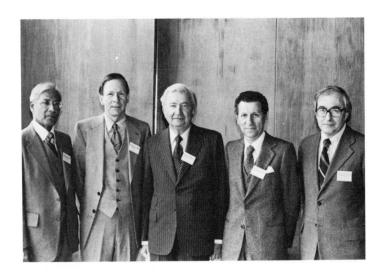

John Sheehan, center, with Ajay
K. Bose (professor of chemistry at
Stevens Institute of Technology
and former graduate student of
Sheehan's at MIT), Gerald Laubach
(international president of Charles
Pfizer, Inc., and former graduate
student of Sheehan's), Murray
Goodman (professor of chemistry
at University of California, San
Diego, and former post-doctoral
fellow of Sheehan's), and Burton
Christensen (director of antibiotics
research at Merck Sharp &
Dohme). The occasion was the
Sheehan Symposium at Stevens
Institute of Technology, March
1980.

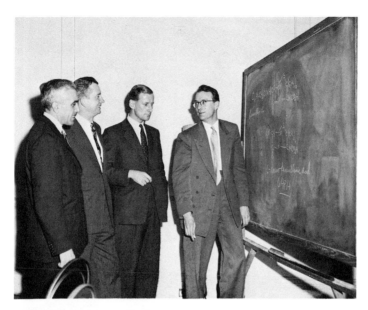

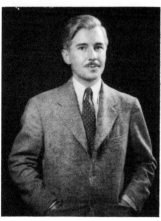

Contemplating the structural formula of 6-aminopenicillanic acid (6-APA) are Amel Menotti, John Sheehan, George Rolinson, and Peter Doyle (Rolinson and Doyle of Beecham at that time) on April 27, 1959. This was just after Beecham published their 6-APA research, during the brief honeymoon period of the Bristol-Beecham penicillin program.

Werner Bachmann, Sheehan's professor at the University of Michigan. Sheehan studied organic synthesis with him and, while a post-doctoral fellow, worked with him on the synthesis of explosive RDX, or cyclonite. In 1943 the CMR recruited Bachmann as a general consultant for the penicillin synthesis program.

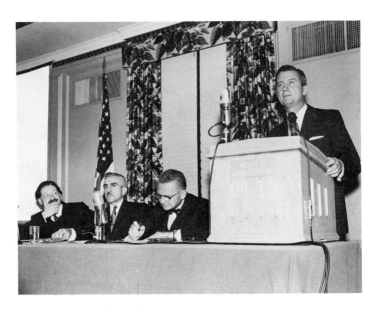

Ernst Chain, Amel Menotti,
Chester Keefer (then professor of
medicine at Boston University
School of Medicine and a consul-
tant for the OSRD), and John
Sheehan at the dedication of the
new research building at Bristol
Laboratories, Syracuse, New York.

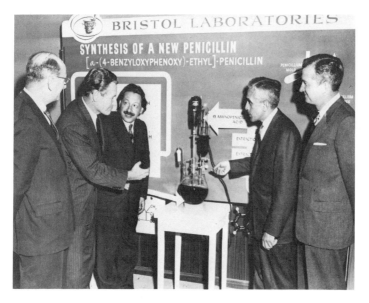

Governor Nelson A. Rockefeller
about to synthesize a new penicillin. Watching are Fred Swartz
(then chairman of the board of
Bristol-Myers), Ernst Chain, Amel
Menotti, and John Sheehan.

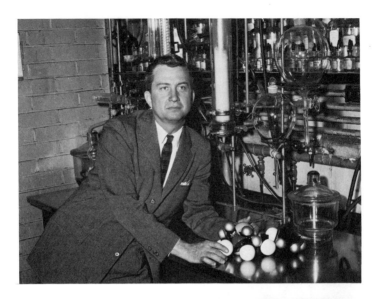

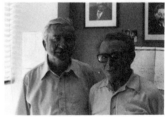

John Sheehan in his laboratory, 1957, holding a model of penicillin. In the background is some of the equipment used in the synthesis of penicillin. The uninitiated are surprised by the simplicity of the laboratory.

John Sheehan and Max Tishler in Professor Tishler's office at Wesleyan University. Tishler was Sheehan's immediate superior at Merck and later became president of Merck Sharp & Dohme Research Laboratories.

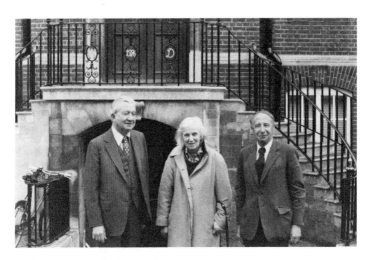

John Sheehan with professor emeritus Dorothy Crowfoot Hodgkin, Nobel Laureate crystallographer who confirmed the structure of penicillin, and Professor Edward Abraham, pioneer in penicillin research and co-discoverer of the cephalosporins. The picture was taken in front of the Sir William Dunn School of Pathology, Oxford, where Abraham, Florey, Chain, and Heatley began their collaborative research on penicillin.

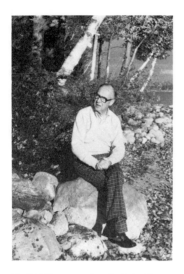

Karl Folkers was head of the Fundamental Research Group at Merck when the company was involved with penicillin.

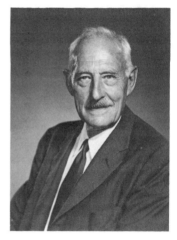

Hans Clarke was one of the directors of the OSRD penicillin program.

# 5  The Conquest of Penicillin

The situation is puzzling and may be unique in the annals of medicinal chemistry that a clinically useful drug showing such prodigious powers as penicillin would be accepted by the medical community and by the pharmaceutical industry essentially in the form nature presented it to them. For a period of approximately eleven years after the close of the massive effort during World War II in 1946, apparently no other laboratory in the world worked on the chemistry of penicillin except my group and I, who worked alone in a set of small laboratories at MIT. One could speculate that in the postwar period it was difficult to obtain financing from industrial or governmental sources for penicillin research. Investigators, at least those in the academic world, were therefore forced to tackle other problems just to keep their research teams together. The pharmaceutical companies, too, had apparently decided that further research on beta-lactam chemistry would not be financially attractive. The naturally fermented penicillins, after all, were more than sufficient to maintain the market. I believe that the general attitude was that the natural penicillins were good enough. To spend any more money on chemical modifications of the antibiotics would only gild the lily. In short, chemists were admonished not to try to improve on nature, or at least not to tamper unnecessarily with the work of the *Penicillium* mold. This same decision had apparently been reached by government funding groups as well. The National Institutes of Health, National Science Foundation, and the Office of

Naval Research, to name but three of the most obvious ones, were no more eager than the commercial firms to support penicillin research.

I can well understand why no major effort was continued on the total synthesis of penicillin. Hundreds of investigators had already spent too much time and effort on the fruitless search for a chemical process that would replace the *Penicillium* mold. It puzzles me, however, that no research program was devoted to chemical modifications of the natural penicillins already isolated. No accounts appeared in the scientific literature to indicate that any serious effort was being made in industry, in academia, or in government laboratories. That statement is true of chemical research worldwide.

The failure to synthesize penicillin and the great difficulty chemists had experienced in even such basic studies as discerning the correct structure of the molecule dissuaded virtually all the experienced research workers from continuing their penicillin research. Younger chemists, who might have been intrigued by the penicillin question and who might have brought fresh insights to the old problem, were probably frightened out of the field by the unhappy experiences of the veterans. Word was out that penicillin was a difficult and sensitive molecule to work with, and prudence dictated that chemists devote themselves to other more amenable problems.

Although the open scientific literature does not reveal any direct attempt on the synthesis of the penicillins during the period immediately after the close of the OSRD penicillin program, one highly placed organic chemist commented to me that he was certain that nearly every big chemical laboratory—and especially the academic laboratories—was making a last attempt at synthesizing penicillins. "Of course they were not publishing," he said. "When they found that their results were no more promising than those obtained during the war program, they simply swallowed their pride and suppressed their research." Rumors also trickled along the professional grapevine that one chemist or another was still tinkering with the penicillin synthesis in his spare time. Adolf Butenandt, the famed German biochemist who had been forbidden by the German government in 1939 from accepting the Nobel Prize for his work on sex hormones, published a small note on his work toward a synthesis of the penicillins. Robert B. Woodward told me that he, too, had tried a new series of penicillin experiments at Harvard, but they led him nowhere. Gilbert Stork at Columbia, Nelson Leonard at the University of Illinois, and others were probably at work. They were all discouraged yet again; no chemist could report significant progress toward the synthesis of penicillins.

The political, economic, and scientific atmosphere in the early 1950s was right to renew enthusiasm for research on the wonder drug, but penicillin had lost the aura with which it had been endowed a decade earlier. In July 1952, the United States Defense Production Administration asked the penicillin producers to increase their output by 140 percent. In preparation for the Korean War, the military had set a goal of 600 trillion units of penicillin per year by January 1, 1955 (*New York Times,* July 15, 1952). The incentive for the pharmaceutical industry was attractive tax write-offs for the necessary capital improvements. But the Korean War did not command the same popular enthusiasm as World War II. Nor was penicillin the high priority item it was during those years of the early 1940s. The head of Pfizer, John E. McKeen, reported that penicillin was no longer their leading product by early 1953. Pfizer, the largest producer of natural penicillins, sold $105 million worth of penicillin in 1952 at prices that had dropped 40 percent by that year. According to McKeen, the leading antibiotic product of the Pfizer line was Terramycin, with sales at $107 million for 1952 and at a stable price (*New York Times,* February 11, 1953).

Early in 1952, the United States Food and Drug Administration and the Atomic Energy Commission sought the interest of sixteen pharmaceutical companies in a pilot project to improve penicillin production by irradiating the mold with gamma rays from cobalt-60. The program would cost less than $100,000 and would save an estimated $5 million a year. But the program depended on whether manufacturers would agree to share the costs of the program. They did not (*New York Times,* February 15, 1952).

In April 1951, I received the American Chemical Society Award in Pure Chemistry for work on the chemistry of the penicillins and peptides. Our synthesis of 5-phenylpenicillin in the MIT laboratories represented substantial progress toward a rational synthesis of the penicillins. We had shown that a penicillin could be synthesized in the laboratory. Unfortunately, the penicillin we had synthesized proved to have no detectable antibiotic properties. It was only a matter of time, once this was done, before we could complete the synthesis of a useful penicillin. Our work was applauded by the *New York Times* (April 5, 1951) as "the closest approach to penicillin by unambiguous methods yet made." The key words in their report are "by unambiguous methods." Unlike earlier chemical approaches to the synthesis of penicillin, we could account for every bond and every chemical process in forging that bond.

In 1956 our laboratory synthesized the chemical nucleus of the penicillin molecule, the ring system we had named 6-aminopenicillanic acid, 6-APA for short. We were then at least within striking distance of acylating it to form a variety of new penicillins. It was clear for the first time in the history of this difficult substance that the penicillin molecule could be modified and manufactured by purely chemical means.

Somewhat later, an entirely different procedure for supplying 6-APA was discovered by the Beecham Laboratories in England. By interfering with the metabolic activities of the *Penicillium* mold, the microorganisms could be made to produce free 6-APA, the chemical nucleus of the penicillin molecule, rather than a penicillin. Both my own work and the Beecham approach could permit the preparation of chemical intermediates of synthetic and semisynthetic penicillins at commercially attractive prices. Suddenly the chemistry of penicillin became a lively research problem again.

Consequently, through the 1960s, a great deal of research into the beta-lactams was renewed in many laboratories throughout the world. In the 1970s and up to the present, research on the beta-lactam antibiotics has increased dramatically. Some estimates are that the worldwide research effort in the beta-lactam antibiotics exceeds several billion dollars a year, by far the largest research and development effort of the present pharmaceutical industry. Coincidentally, the discovery of cephalosporin C in 1953 by Abraham and Newton, furthermore, pointed the way to a whole class of new antibiotics containing the seemingly magical beta-lactam ring.

I do not know of any parallel case in which interest in a compound or family of compounds has gone through such a dramatic rise and fall. One could point to morphine, perhaps, as another example. For at least a hundred years efforts have been made to find derivatives of morphine that preserve the strong analgesic properties of the group but without the addicting side effects. Morphine research continues to the present day. That research, however, has never reached the high intensity that characterized the penicillin work during the war, nor does it compare with the magnitude of the research effort continuing today.

### Predictions of Success
I was determined not to give up on the penicillin problem. True I thought massive expenditures of time and money had failed to solve the problem; but, on the other hand, the failures and limited successes carefully recorded in the thousands of pages of PEN Reports during the OSRD

project could lead an enterprising and patient chemist to the ultimate goal. I also recognized that the important difference between the OSRD penicillin synthesis program and my own research agenda was time. Given enough time to sift through the many reports, to think about the problem, and to try new approaches, sooner or later I would come up with a workable solution.

The problem of financial support was solved with remarkable ease. Dr. Amel Menotti, who was director of research at Bristol at the time, was looking for an academic organic chemist to serve as consultant to his group. We were introduced by the late Arthur Cope. Professor Cope had been one of the most promising young chemists of his time and later became an influential member of the scientific community. He was always a strong supporter of young chemists in all fields. I am proud to say that Arthur Cope provided not only material support for my budding career but that he also served as an inspiration. From him I learned that one can successfully keep several projects going at the same time. Professor Cope, for instance, at one point had more than twenty graduate students, was president of the American Chemical Society, conducted his own research, and was department head at MIT. And, with all this to occupy his attention, he made the effort to introduce Amel Menotti and me. Almost from our first meeting Menotti and I had close rapport. We decided that I would consult on a number of problems and eventually offer Bristol what help I could on the production of penicillin. I am sure that Bristol was particularly interested in me because of my five years' experience in the pharmaceutical industry at Merck. That work had given me a feel for how pharmaceutical laboratories attack their chemical problems. Purely academic chemists, lacking this experience in industry, might not have served the needs of Bristol so well.

Bristol and I quickly agreed upon a mutually advantageous arrangement. I would serve as consultant to Bristol

Laboratories and Bristol would support some of my penicillin research.

Our arrangement worked out well for both of us: Bristol supported my penicillin research from 1948 to 1970. Their support was more than financial. During the most important years of my penicillin synthesis research, Bristol Laboratories carried out the necessary microbiological assays of the chemical products I developed and supplied me with many of the chemical intermediates needed for the syntheses.

In addition to the formal support I received from Bristol, I enjoyed considerable help from Merck and Company. Although we had no formal arrangement Merck supplied me with critical intermediates. This courtesy was arranged by Max Tishler in particular.

I had several reasons for continuing the penicillin research where so many had failed before me. It was clear to me that the last word had not yet been said in the matter. Of course the natural penicillins were a great success; but I was certain that knowing more about the chemical properties of the penicillins would allow, if not the complete synthesis, at least the chemical alteration of penicillin in ways that might well prove beneficial. We would learn about penicillin itself and, perhaps, learn about the living systems that synthesize the penicillins and similar beta-lactam compounds. I had hoped, naturally, that my work on penicillin would lead to an eventual synthesis. The scientific importance of synthesizing such a compound that had baffled the best chemists of a generation was a great incentive, for I knew that someone would solve the problem eventually. I wanted to be that person.

In a talk I gave at the organic synthesis symposium in Ann Arbor, Michigan, in the early 1950s, I described some of the plans I had been making for future work on penicillin. I predicted five clinically significant properties of penicillin that could be enhanced in a chemically altered penicillin. At least four of these predictions have now been fully realized;

work is progressing on the fifth. It is unusual in pharmaceutical research to be able to predict the properties of new compounds with this high degree of accuracy. But so much chemical work had been done on the penicillins that I felt confident about the scientific evidence on which each prediction was founded.

My first prediction was that a new penicillin could be developed with increased acid stability. It was reasonably well known that natural penicillin was easily inactivated by the acid in the stomach. In the presence of acid, penicillin goes to penillic acid, probably through an oxazolone type of intermediate. That troublesome rearrangement and degradation had been one of the major stumbling blocks throughout the chemical history of penicillin. If one were to design a synthetic penicillin in which the side chain could form an oxazolone, the newly designed molecule would show greater resistance to acid. What effect this chemical change would have on the biological activity of the new penicillin was impossible to know in advance. But I thought that finding a biologically active compound that had the right side chain to prevent acid inactivation was possible.

My second prediction was that the microbiological spectrum of a synthetic penicillin could be broader than that of any natural penicillin. As Fleming observed in his initial experiments with penicillin in 1928, the natural penicillins were active against Gram-positive microorganisms—staphylococci, streptococci, pneumococci, and so forth—but not against Gram-negative microorganisms—*Escherichia coli* and the salmonellas, including those responsible for typhoid. I thought that if the penicillin molecule were altered substantially, starting with modifications of the side chain and perhaps even changing features of the penicillin nucleus itself, one might be able to change properties of the compound so that a synthetic penicillin would be produced that was effective against Gram-negative organisms.

Why natural penicillins are effective only against Gram-positive microorganisms is still not known. Nevertheless, it was a good guess at the time that if one changed the electrolyte properties of the molecule, for example, by introducing a basic function, this chemical change would affect the transport of penicillin through the bacterial cell wall and might lead to greater activity of penicillin against Gram-negative microorganisms. As if nature were actively encouraging this line of reasoning, penicillin N, which was shown to have an amino group (that is, a basic function) on the side chain, did show marked activity against the Gram-negative microorganisms. This promising lead was later exploited in penicillin research and led to the development of ampicillin, one of the first and still one of the most successful broad-spectrum antibiotics. Still later, the discovery of cephalosporin C, a new type of naturally occurring beta-lactam antibiotic, confirmed the hypothesis that a basic function on the side chain could make an antibiotic effective against Gram-negative microorganisms.

Third, I was certain that activity against penicillin-resistant organisms could be enhanced. One mechanism of penicillin resistance had been discovered and elaborated in many laboratories. Abraham's group at Oxford was one of the first to describe the role of certain enzymes produced by the microorganisms in the inactivation of penicillin. Resistance to penicillin is due to the ability of some microorganisms to produce the enzyme penicillinase, which opens the beta-lactam ring. Opening the beta-lactam ring inactivates the penicillin and so the microorganisms are no longer victims of its antibiotic power. Penicillins kill bacteria by interrupting metabolic processes responsible for building the cell wall of the microorganisms. Because animal cells have no comparable cell wall, penicillin is highly specific against bacteria and is virtually nontoxic to cells of the animal host. In the presence of penicillinase, even high concentrations of penicillin leave the bacterial cell wall unharmed. This resistance presented a major problem in the outbreaks of "house staff" that plagued hospitals in the early days of penicillin treatment.

Microbiologists later learned that microbes have at least two other lines of resistance to penicillin. Some microorganisms produce another enzyme, known as amidase, which is capable of cutting the amide bond that attaches the side chain of the penicillin molecule to the 6-APA nucleus. As with penicillinase, this enzymatic destruction of the penicillin molecule also destroys its antibiotic properties. As a third defense some microorganisms apparently develop a genetic trait that allows them to resist penicillin. Once they have developed this trait, they can transmit it to their offspring.

It seemed to me in the early 1950s that a chemist should be able to alter the penicillin molecule so that a synthetic penicillin retained the ability to inhibit formation of the cell wall and yet would not be destroyed by the defensive enzymes of the microorganism. These are two quite different properties, and so, I thought, it should be possible to design a molecule capable of doing one without affecting the other.

One of the more obvious ways to make the penicillin molecule impervious to the action of penicillinase would be to protect the beta-lactam. One way of providing this protection would be to increase the steric hindrance around the beta-lactam so that the penicillinase would not bind so easily to its active site on the penicillin molecule. I realized that finding the right protective groups might not be simple because the bulky groups needed to protect the beta-lactam could not be so large that they would interfere with the desired ability of the penicillin to inhibit cell wall formation. One of the products of this line of reasoning, staphcillin, has two methoxyl groups that crowd around the beta-lactam function so that it is well protected from attack by penicillinase. Methicillin, the oxacillins, and a number of other synthetic penicillins have now been developed for this purpose.

RCO$_2$H + H $\quad$ H

6-Aminopenicillanic acid
(6-APA)

hydrolysis

Site of amidase action

Site of
penicillinase action

Penicilloic acid

Site of action by penicillinase and amidase.

Fourth, I thought that allergenicity could be minimized in a synthetic penicillin. From very early in the history of penicillin, the most serious side effect of the drug has been its ability to sensitize some patients. Although only a small proportion of people taking penicillin develop allergic reactions, for this minority penicillin can be a life-threatening poison instead of a life-saving drug. Whether the allergenicity is due to penicillin itself or to impurities introduced in the preparation of the drug had not been clarified. According to Dr. Gordon Stewart, a highly purified penicillin would not be allergenic because the allergic response is due to protein impurities carried along from the original fermentation of wholly natural penicillins or from the enzymatic removal of the side chains in the preparation of semisynthetic penicillins. If Stewart were right, the newer synthetic penicillins and the cephalosporins would not produce allergic responses in penicillin-sensitive patients.

When I prepared totally synthetic penicillin V, very early in our own synthetic work, I realized that allergenicity is a property of the penicillin molecule itself. This totally synthetic penicillin, which had never seen any fermentation broth, still produced allergic responses in certain penicillin-sensitive patients.

The allergic response, however, could be minimized by administering the drug orally. Perhaps more important, if a serious allergic response did develop after oral administration of penicillin, the problem could be rectified more easily than if the penicillin were administered endermically. An offending substance can be removed more easily from the digestive tract than from the blood stream and tissues. There have been attempts to use penicillinase as an antidote for penicillin in cases of severe allergic reaction, but this procedure has not been entirely successful. Because the body is exquisitely sensitive to even the smallest amount of some offending substance, the penicillinase antidote would have to reduce the penicillin concentration to an exceedingly low level.

Finally, I was certain when I made my predictions, that greater horsepower could be built into a synthetic penicillin molecule. I felt strongly that new penicillins could be designed with better oral absorption, less serum binding, slower excretion, and so forth so that more of the administered penicillin would destroy the microorganisms and less would be tied up by the body or excreted from it.

For all these reasons, I felt in the late 1940s and early 1950s that the chemists had not yet had the last word on penicillin. I knew that important work remained to be done on the natural and synthetic penicillins. And I set out to do some of that work.

### A New Way to Make Peptide Bonds

As is customary when a research scientist leaves an industrial laboratory, Merck and Company asked me to refrain from doing any more work on the projects I had been involved with while at their laboratory. We had made good progress at Merck on the production and isolation of penicillin. Naturally, if I were to continue this work on my own, I might conceivably have jeopardized Merck's position.

As a result, when I arrived at MIT I worked on problems of peptide chemistry and not problems directly related to penicillin, although there was some connection between the two. The peptide bond, linking the amide and carboxylic groups of adjacent amino acids, is the general family of bonds to which the beta-lactam belongs. In a formal sense, the peptide bond involves the abstraction of the elements of water from the amine and the carboxyl group of two amino acids by joining the hydroxyl group of the carboxyl function with the hydrogen (or proton) of the amine function. This coupling is shown more easily with a picture of what is sometimes derisively known as lasso chemistry.

$$R-\overset{O}{\overset{\|}{C}} + HN-R' \rightarrow R-\overset{O}{\overset{\|}{C}}-N-R' + H_2O$$

Schematic diagram of peptide bond formation.

Water is formed as a by-product of this reaction, and the amino and carboxyl groups are coupled to form a peptide. This process of peptide formation takes place in almost all living organisms, for wherever proteins and other peptidelike substances are made, they are made by this general reaction. By learning more about the chemical properties of peptide bonds in general and by learning more about how to synthesize these vital compounds, I thought we just might learn more about the synthesis of penicillin.

I had been thinking about the formation of peptide bonds in chemical and physiological systems and felt that thermodynamic considerations argued against the reactions normally given in biology to describe how peptide bonds were formed in the assembly of protein molecules. It seemed more likely, rather, that a lower-energy system could be devised in the laboratory and that this set of reactions would probably be a better model of what happens under physiological conditions than the reactions normally given in the textbooks.

I realized that we needed a special reagent for this work, a reagent with particular properties that hitherto had not been combined in a single chemical compound. The requirements were dictated by the idiosyncracies of penicillin: The new reagent must tolerate an aqueous environment; it must form peptide bonds under relatively mild conditions; and it must work fairly rapidly.

For a number of years prior to the 1950s, I had felt that there should be a way of forming a peptide bond in fully aqueous solutions. I pointed out to some of my colleagues in biochemistry that nature does this all the time. Although enzymes seem to possess magical properties, even enzymatic activity must ultimately be explicable as an ordinary chemical reaction. Enzymes, too, must follow the laws of organic chemistry.

The carboxyl group was the obvious one to activate. Many ways of activating it for reaction with an amino group were already available to the organic chemist. For example, an acid chloride or anhydride might be used to join the amino and carboxyl groups of adjacent molecules. The acid chlorides, however, may be sensitive to moisture. Some may even react explosively with water and would clearly not be appropriate for the penicillin reaction I was designing. Others may react more slowly with water, but even these acid chlorides and anhydrides possessed unwanted properties that made them unsuitable for the penicillin work. Because penicillin could not tolerate acid conditions, acid chlorides were clearly out of the question. An acid chloride might not be an acid itself but, in reacting to form the peptide, it would release HCl, which would produce an acid in the aqueous conditions of our intended penicillin reaction. I needed a reagent that was not only neutral itself but one that did not produce acidic products.

I searched for a reagent that would add to the carboxyl group to form a reactive intermediate and yet would not react with molecular water at appreciable speeds. I had hoped that this ideal reagent would survive for hours or even days in water and, if an amine were present, would nevertheless acylate the amine. This was a tall order. No such reagent was known at the time. But although I could not immediately order it from the storeroom, I could at least simplify my search by describing the requirements of this reagent.

One Sunday afternoon, as I was reading through some of my back journals, I chanced upon an article on the preparation of an obscure class of compounds known as carbodiimides. Because the carbodiimides could readily abstract the elements of water, these compounds had been used, to some extent, as drying agents in certain highly specialized applications. Alexander Todd, for instance, had used them in the preparation of pyrophosphates. Although the chemical literature did not mention using carbodiimides to make an amide bond, their ability to abstract the elements of water made them instantly attractive to me for use in the peptide work. The current literature was unanimous, however, in warning that the carbodiimides were extremely sensitive to water. That surely would militate against using them in the aqueous conditions preferred for the penicillin synthesis.

The article I happened upon that Sunday afternoon changed my thinking about the carbodiimides. It described the standard recipe for preparing dicyclohexylcarbodiimide (DCC) by treating a thiourea with lead oxide and then swirling the mixture for hours or even days. The function of the lead oxide is to abstract the elements of hydrogen sulfide from the thiourea, thereby forming the carbodiimide. The chemical reaction for preparing dicyclohexylcarbodiimide (DCC) I used in my original work is

$$\underset{\substack{\text{Dicyclohexyl-}\\\text{thiourea}}}{C_6H_{11}NH\overset{\overset{\displaystyle S}{\|}}{C}NHC_6H_{11}} + \underset{\text{Lead Oxide}}{PbO} \rightarrow \underset{\substack{\text{Dicyclohexyl-}\\\text{carbodiimide}\\(DCC)}}{C_6H_{11}N{=}C{=}NC_6H_{11}} + \underset{\substack{\text{Lead}\\\text{Sulfide}}}{PbS} + \underset{\text{Water}}{H_2O}$$

Preparation of dicyclohexylcarbodiimide (DCC).

As I read through the familiar reactions that Sunday, I saw with a shock of recognition that in the process of making DCC, the elements of water are also produced. That meant that for two whole days, a carbodiimide could exist in the presence of a full molar equivalent of water. It meant that the carbodiimides could not be as sensitive to molecular water as had been suggested by all the earlier reviews.

The next day I went into the laboratory to meet with George Hess, one of my post-doctoral fellows. George had received his doctoral degree from the University of California, Berkeley, for work with Professor C. H. Li on adrenocorticotropic hormone. He had also done some biochemical work. In February 1953, George wrote to me, asking if he could join my laboratory. "At this time, I would like to have more training in organic chemistry and peptide synthesis. In addition to some formal training in organic chemistry, including a laboratory course in organic chemistry, I have had very little actual laboratory experience. I have synthesized two dipeptides by the carbobenzoxy-chloride method and a few DNP [dinitrophenyl] amino acids. I am now applying for two post-doctoral fellowships" (February 9, 1953). George was awarded a fellowship by the National Foundation for Infantile Paralysis and so he came to me with his own research money. We began work in the fall of 1953.

The method I had worked out for coupling two blocked amino acids was to use a thiol acid, that is, an acid in which the −OH group has been replaced by the −SH group. It had been known at the time that such thiol acids did form amides from carboxylic acids and amines. I had hoped that the hydrogen sulfide would be evolved more readily than the water to form the peptide bond. The application of this technique had been proceeding rather slowly. When I came upon the idea of using a carbodiimide as the coupling agent, I thought of George as the logical person to try it out. He had the materials, he had some experience, and it seemed appropriate at the time to change the direction of his research.

I suggested to George that he take an amino-blocked amino acid and a carboxyl-blocked peptide, add an equivalent of carbodiimide in a solvent such as methylene chloride, and see what would happen. Since my laboratory was already working on peptides, we had several samples of peptides and intermediates available in the laboratory, some that we had made ourselves and others available from other research groups. Some of the peptides were optically active. We were doubly fortunate in having some DCC reagent available, too. (Dicyclohexylcarbodiimide became commercially available in 1959 from the Peirce Chemical Company (Ferris deposition, p. 16), but it was still an esoteric reagent and not readily found in laboratory storerooms.)

George treated the amino acid and the peptide with the

DCC and within an hour came back to my office full of excitement. "It is very strange," he said. "A solid is precipitating out quickly, and this is happening at room temperature."

"Wait until no more solid seems to be forming," I said, "and then separate the solid. We can identify that product and then see what remains in the solvent."

When no more solid was forming, he then filtered and washed the solid to remove impurities and identified the precipitate. He found dicyclohexylurea. Water had been removed from the molecules of the amine and carboxylic acid. When George concentrated the product dissolved in methylene chloride and allowed that product to crystallize, he found that he had indeed synthesized a peptide under mild conditions. The yield was impressively high considering the difficulties chemists had experienced with bonds of this sort.

We found it difficult to monitor precisely the rate of this reaction because the urea tends to supersaturate the solution rather than to precipitate directly as the reaction proceeds. Consequently, observing the precipitation of urea as a measure of when the reaction is complete is a bit like listening to the thunder to find out when the lightning stroke is complete. Nevertheless we could be sure that at room temperature the carbodiimide coupling was complete in less than four hours.

The bonds from a carbon atom form a four-sided pyramid, with the carbon atom at the center. If all four of the groups attached to a single carbon atom are different from each other, two different arrangements of the constituents are possible. The carbon is said to be chiral (that is, "handed"), and the mirror image of this asymmetric arrangement will not be superimposable on the original. The classic analogy is the right- and left-handed glove. Each member of the pair of D,L configurations is known as an antipode, and usually each has different physiological properties. We were quite relieved to learn, therefore, that our reaction with carbodiimide did not racemize the product.

George and I published an account of our work. "We wish to describe a new and very useful method of forming peptide or other amide bonds. Two components, one containing a free carboxyl function and the other a free amino group, couple directly and rapidly with high yield on treatment with N,N'-dicyclohexylcarbodiimide at room temperature." The paper caused a sensation. According to one commentator, "Dicyclohexylcarbodiimide has become the most widely used activating agent in peptide synthesis. Virtually every solid phase synthesis and many solution syntheses employ DCC, either directly or through the use of active esters" (Daniel H. Rich and Jasbir Singh in *The Peptides,* Erhard Gross and Johannes Meinhofer, eds. [New York: Academic Press, 1979], p. 242). More than 80 percent of peptide syntheses reported in the literature after publication of our paper employed the carbodiimide method. The paper itself is one of the most often cited research reports in the history of chemistry.

### Experimenting with DCC

Use of carbodiimide as a coupling agent gave me an important clue to how I might close a beta-lactam ring. Essentially all familiar methods of making amides had already been tried in the effort to synthesize penicillin during World War II, and all those efforts to close the beta-lactam ring failed. The only possible exception to this statement is the work by du Vigneaud to fuse an oxazolone and thiazolidine according to the old mistaken Robinson formula. The yield of the du Vigneaud reaction was low, but the real criticism of that work is that there was no possible way of improving the yield. The synthesis was totally misdirected. The carbodiimide reagent, on the other hand, seemed for the first time to give chemists a way of closing the beta-lactam ring according to a rationally planned synthesis, directed by the correct beta-lactam formula for penicillin.

Penicillin, as we knew, was highly sensitive to acid and base. DCC is neutral, and the reaction products are neutral, too. Penicillin is highly sensitive to degradation by high temperature. Carbodiimide reacted with the carboxyl and amino groups quickly to form a peptide bond and the reaction proceeded at or below room temperature. Finally, carbodiimide would react in an aqueous solution best suited for penicillin synthesis. All in all, it appeared that in carbodiimide I had found the ideal reagent for closing the beta-lactam and, eventually, for completing that last troublesome step in the synthesis of penicillin.

The precise mechanism by which peptide bonds are formed is not well understood even at present. Most chemists believe that the reaction is endergonic, that is, that the reaction requires the input of energy for it to proceed. In natural systems, this energy is supplied by the universal fuel of cells, adenosine triphosphate (ATP). Breaking one of the high-energy phosphate bonds to yield adenosine diphosphate (ADP) releases energy, which the cell can use to drive its own metabolic processes. My colleagues in biochemistry, revealing their own vitalist prejudices, said that I would not be able to produce a similar reaction in the laboratory. "You will not be able to carry out that reaction without an energy source," they said, "one like the complicated system of metabolic reactions that transfers the energy from the ATP to the particular chemical reaction to be powered by it in the cell."

In general, a reaction will not proceed unless, as we say, it is going downhill thermodynamically. In other words, energy must ultimately be released in the process. There may be an energy barrier to overcome, by heating or by the adept use of catalysts, but in the end, the products of the reaction must have a lower heat of combustion than the reagents. In the case of the carbodiimide reactions, some of the driving force of the reaction may be liberated in the process by which the carbodiimide goes to urea. There is a hydration of the molecule, and that almost certainly supplies some of the energy required by the reaction to form the peptide bond. What the biochemists failed to recognize, however, is that the carbodiimide itself acts as the energy source.

An obviously difficult question to answer is why the carbodiimide is so stable at pHs of approximately 7 in the presence of a large excess of water but will nevertheless very rapidly—sometimes in a matter of seconds—take the elements of water from the carboxylic acid and the amine. In some experiments that I have reported, especially studies of the water-soluble carbodiimides, I allowed the water-soluble carbodiimide to stand for a period of forty-eight hours. I then removed the water by freeze-drying and tested the purity of the carbodiimide by melting point, infrared spectrum, and by other means. I could not measure a change in the carbodiimide.

Perhaps the carbodiimide remains unchanged in the presence of water because of the formation of an O-acylurea—that is, the acyl group is on the oxygen. Being an anhydride it would be expected to react quickly with an amine if the amine is present in sufficient concentration. It does not react with the molecular water at pH 7. If there is not an amine present, or if there is a trace of tertiary amine, there is rearrangement to the N-acylurea, and that compound is not an acylating agent. No one has been able to isolate O-acylurea. I did not suggest this mechanism in any of our papers because I did not have any direct or even indirect evidence for such a mechanism or for the presence of this intermediate, but some of my colleagues have suggested this as a possible explanation.

The discovery of the carbodiimides offered us a promising lead, but I was still not out of the woods. We began to have difficulties with our carbodiimide reactions. Even in attempting to reproduce his own experiments, George Hess found that his laboratory results were erratic. To my chagrin, we occasionally found significant yields of racemized product, changing the optical and physiological properties of the peptides we were synthesizing. Sometimes, too, we found unexpected and unwanted side products of the reaction. To make matters worse, I began hearing from other laboratories around the country that they, too, were having difficulties with our published procedure. No one, not even our own group, could reproduce our synthesis of peptides with DCC reliably.

Our habits of careful research, however, paid off. After considerable experimentation, I identified the source of the trouble. It is generally thought that the active intermediate in this reaction is a compound involving the carbodiimide and the carboxyl group. I found that in the presence of even a trace of base this crucial intermediate can rearrange to yield the unwanted products we were detecting. As the reaction environment is made more basic, more of the undesired rearrangement occurs. Changes in the solvent, too, affected the racemization, especially in the presence of basic solvents.

Our original laboratory instructions called for equal molar equivalents of all three reagents—the carbodiimide, the carboxyl-bearing molecule, and the amine-bearing molecule. Our directions were correct in theory but impossible in practice because of the sheer magnitude of Avogadro's number. This number, equal to the number of molecules in a molar equivalent of a compound is an unimaginable $6.02 \times 10^{23}$. In other words, a mole of water, which weighs 18 grams, will contain $6.02 \times 10^{23}$ molecules. Even the most sensitive balance cannot weigh strictly equal amounts of the reagents. The actual number of molecules can differ by several orders of magnitude. In most chemical reactions, this slight imprecision is tolerable. In the case of our carbodiimide reactions, on the other hand, because they were so sensitive to even the slightest excess of base, the imprecision was enough to make success of the carbodiimide reaction a hit or miss affair.

Science cannot tolerate random success. The trick was therefore to find a way of guaranteeing that the disastrous excess of base did not occur in the reaction. The solution to our problem, once I recognized this simple fact, was no more complicated than being sure that the instructions called for a slight excess of the acid-bearing molecule in the reaction. With this slight alteration in the experimental instructions, most of the problems disappeared.

In recalling my work on this reaction, a former student Istvan Lengyel, commented that my DCC peptide synthesis had been a great surprise to the European peptide chemists with whom he had been working. They had been using the classical peptide techniques. His own teacher, Professor Bruckner, very formal and impressive as so many European academics of that generation were, was among the most dazzled. He obviously imparted some of his own respect for my chemical feat to his student, for when Istvan finally came to study with me at MIT, he told me that he was surprised indeed to find that the chemist who had revolutionized peptide chemistry in Europe was hardly older than he was. He said that he was even more amazed to find that the chemist who had shaken peptide chemistry to its foundations, even had a sense of humor.

Ajay Bose, one of my graduate students at the time, had a similar impression.

At that time, Sheehan was quite young, barely 30, and some of the students who were veterans of the Second World War were not much younger than him; so there was not that distance that you would expect to find in the Old World or in Europe. As a matter of fact, coming as I do from India, I was rather shocked at this intimacy between the Herr Professor and his students. But Sheehan was considered to be one of the pleasant and affable types of professors and not inaccessible or cold. . . .

I was at MIT during the period 1947 through 1950, and at

that time Professor Sheehan's group was not as large as it got to be later. There were about ten Ph.D. students and one post-doctoral at that time, I seem to recall, and Professor Sheehan was quite easily accessible. He had to go through the corridor to go to his own office, which was right opposite our laboratory, and it was quite customary for him at that time to stop in the laboratory quite often—not on any particularly regular basis at a preset time, but at different times he would come into the laboratory and talk to different people. And we too would go see him. We didn't have to make an appointment to see him; we could go knock on his door and talk to him if he were free or if we had something that needed clarification. On the other hand, if we had found something quite exciting, we didn't hesitate to go barge into his office and tell him about it. . . .

He was always interested in knowing what new factors had emerged or what new points of view had come out in the course of the work that was going on and would have to make written reports, if I remember correctly, once at the end of each term. But other than that there were a number of occasions where one would have to go fairly in detail about what he was doing. There were different occasions when one would have to go to Professor Sheehan of necessity. For example, every time we made a new compound we certainly would like to get an analysis done on it, and those days, the analyst would not touch our compound unless we had filled in the form and we had Professor Sheehan's signature on it. Of course, if we went to see him to get his signature, he would always ask how did the reaction go and what happened. We had to spend a little time going over the related reactions or other things that might come up during the discussion. We had to go to him if we wanted infrared spectra, again we needed a signature on a form to get that [Bose deposition, pp. 41, 36, 37].

My primary goal at this point was the synthesis of penicillin, but I took a few amusing side trips with the carbodiimide reactions, for I knew that in DCC I had a reagent that would allow me to do many interesting tricks with proteins. Collagen seemed to be an obvious protein to work with. It is used extensively in biological work and can be obtained in pure form. There is a lot of information about this biologically important substance. Once I decided that I would work with collagen, I told one of my colleagues about the series of experiments I was planning and I asked him if he would be able to give me some collagen. He said that he could spare some. This turned out to be several strands of kangaroo tail collagen—kangaroo tail is the staple source of collagen for many biological supply houses. Biologists, as a result, were familiar with kangaroo tail as an experimental substance. My colleagues in chemistry, however, thought that I must have been pretty close to the bottom of the barrel to be devoting my research time to a study of the caudal appendage of the kangaroo.

Nevertheless, my chemical results were excellent. One of my triumphs was a gelatin dessert that would not liquefy in heat. Gelatin is partially degraded collagen. It sets under refrigeration because hydrogen bonds cross link to oxygen atoms of the adjacent gelatin molecules. These bonds are thermally labile; they break when heat gives the physical system more energy. Adding a small amount of carbodiimide to the gelatin changes the bonds from the relatively weak hydrogen bonds to the stronger amide bonds. Treated in this way, gelatin no longer liquefies at warm temperatures.

Another application of the carbodiimide reagent was to the curing of leather and other protein substances. I compared carbodiimide curing with the three standard methods for tanning leather—the chrome-alum, formaldehyde, and glyoxal methods. Results with the carbodiimide were as good as those obtained with the standard methods. The chrome-alum method is the least expensive and could be reserved for the most routine tanning tasks. Formaldehyde and other tanning methods, on the other hand, are used for specialized applications. For example, formaldehyde was used at one point to treat viruses in the preparation of polio vaccine. There is, however, an unfortunate shortcoming of the formaldehyde curing of protein: in aqueous solutions, the formaldehyde reaction is reversed. Some of the viruses treated with formaldehyde revived. I had thought that carbodiimide would cure the virus protein more effectively in the preparation of vaccines, but I did not take this idea beyond the planning stages.

Another idea I actually did test in my laboratory involved conventional home and professional hair curling solutions, which depend on the breaking and remaking of disulfide linkages between the protein molecules of hair. The chemical reagent used in the Toni process is ammonium thioglycolate, a substance that can reduce the disulfide bond. While the bonds are broken, the hair is arranged on curlers, reorienting the disulfide bonds. Adding a solution of ammonium bromate to reconstitute the disulfide bonds imparts the desired curl to the hair. My idea was to use the carbodiimide to form linkages that were stronger than the disulfide bonds. I mentioned this process in the patent I took out on the carbodiimide reagent.

Perhaps my most serious application of carbodiimide reactions was in the preparation of natural surgical sutures. Self-dissolving surgical sutures are usually made from sheep gut. Treating the collagen of the sheep gut with carbodiimide would allow the chemist to create sutures that would dissolve inside the body at precisely controlled rates. The degree of curing with carbodiimide would accurately control the physical characteristics of the suture. If the surgeon wanted a suture that would last for several weeks, for instance, he could choose one type of cured-collagen product. If he wanted a suture that would dissolve within only a few days, he could choose another. Carbodiimide, I found, did not make the suture toxic because nothing was added to the compound; and such products would be completely acceptable for medical use.

My process was investigated by the Ethicon branch of Johnson & Johnson. They reported that they had no trouble in reproducing my work and that the carbodiimide-treated collagen was an excellent material for surgical sutures. But they also told me that they were not going to adopt my process. To do so would have required that they completely retool their manufacturing operation, which at that time depended on the familiar chrome-alum curing technique. They also already had the confidence of surgeons, who had been buying their standard products for years. In fact, when I approached them, the Ethicon branch controlled about 90 percent of the suture market. There was no good reason for them to change their way of manufacturing sutures. And so the idea more or less died on the vine.

The real point of my work, however, was penicillin synthesis. And this work went forward with remarkable success.

### The Synthesis of Penicillin
In organic chemistry there are many surprises and many disappointments; there are no miracles. The laws of chemistry describe the predictable behaviors of compounds. When appropriate conditions are devised, a reproducible reaction will take place. Neither Satan nor anyone else takes the time to mess up the reactions of organic chemists.

By the mid-1950s I had assembled many of the basic tools I needed for the synthesis of penicillin. I had found an exquisitely delicate and selective coupling agent in the carbodiimides. All my experimentation led me to believe that this coupling agent would prove to be the key to the synthesis that had eluded so many chemists in the past. The total synthesis of penicillin finally seemed to be within my grasp.

Several problems remained, however, before I could complete the total synthesis of penicillin. But, as it turned out, these were more or less routine problems, at least compared to those that had blocked progress in the past. The three-dimensional orientation, stereo-isomerism, as we have already seen, would be a major problem in the synthesis of penicillin if the synthesis resulted in a mixture of physiologically different racemates. I needed to learn more about the stereochemistry of penicillin. Although I was certainly not going into large-scale production of penicillin in the preliminary laboratory work, I would nevertheless require kilogram quantities of critical intermediates for the experimental syntheses. Max Tishler of Merck and Amel Menotti of Bristol were very helpful in this regard. Funding was also a problem. But Bristol was always generous with money, materials, and manpower. Bristol, for example, performed the bioassays of my chemical products. Because my penicillin work had the strong support of Professor Cope, chairman of the chemistry department, MIT furnished the necessary space and laboratory facilities.

The most important elements in my research were the people. I was fortunate in having an excellent team of graduate students and post-doctoral fellows: E. J. Corey, Gerald D. Laubach, Ajay Bose, Ken Henery-Logan, David L. Johnson, Philip A. Cruikshank, and many others worked diligently through the years of trial and frustration.

The workshop I assembled was not fancy. I used to refer to it as our Mom and Pop lab. There were a few benches and the usual glassware and equipment. My office was connected with the laboratory that Henery-Logan and I used along with several technicians. Ken Henery-Logan, as my senior post-doctoral fellow, was given charge of the routine laboratory responsibilities. It was so arranged that when I went out one of the two doors to my office—the one I would go out 99 percent of the time—I would walk right past Henery-Logan's desk and past the laboratory where he was working. I buzzed in and out frequently. And as I went through the laboratory, I would stop and talk with either Henery-Logan or the other post-doctoral fellows about how things were going. I made the rounds of my laboratories approximately twice a day, early in the morning and then again late in the afternoon. My standing joke was that you could tell whether a scientist was interested in his research or in the mechanics and politics of the field by whether he first went through his laboratory or through his mail. I went through my laboratories first.

"In 1951, early January, I joined Dr. Sheehan's group as a post-doctoral fellow," said Henery-Logan.

I was very interested in the work on penicillins he was doing. And actually, he had funds only for one post-doctoral fellow who was leaving July the first, so I worked without salary for the first six months and then was put on salary July the first, 1951, and stayed in Dr. Sheehan's group until September of 1960. . . . The duties were connected with all research and, specifically, on the penicillin project in various forms throughout my tenure there. . . . The general instructions I had were that we wanted to make Dr. Sheehan a natural penicillin first [by] whatever manner possible. And subsequently, it was hoped that a method could be devised, not only to make the natural penicillin, but new penicillins that might have improved properties. This was the general instructions I had. I worked on essentially an extension of this same work that was published. At that time, we knew very little about the stereochemistry. And in the condensation reactions that Dave Johnson had carried out first, it turned out to be a mixture of stereoisomers, and he had not separated them at the acid stage [Henery-Logan deposition, April 14, 1977].

Johnson and Cruickshank also had this problem, and the alpha, or natural, series of esters were separated, but not in the acid form.

Henery-Logan described his work further as "cleaning up, sort of a loose end, where the structures had not been established, compounds had been obtained, but the structures had not been established. . . . During this period, I also tried to improve the cyclization reaction" (Henery-Logan deposition, April 14, 1977).

The term *synthesis* is a rather confusing one to the layman as well as to the professional chemist. It can mean many things to many people. In general, there are at least four kinds of synthesis: biosynthesis, partial synthesis, relay synthesis, and total synthesis. I had been interested only in using methods of organic chemistry to arrive at a total synthesis of penicillin without resorting to the products of living organisms at any stage in the synthesis. In synthesizing 6-APA and penicillin itself, for instance, I never used any products of fermentation, enzymes, or other biological substances. My synthesis was all done by using chemicals from the shelf.

The design of the experiment was simple. My research goal, at this point, was to show that DCC could close the beta-lactam ring and that this ring closure could be effected under conditions so mild that they did not disturb the rest of the penicillin molecule. The problem was therefore to design a relay synthesis starting with natural penicillin V, opening and closing the ring, and comparing the final chemical product with the original natural product.

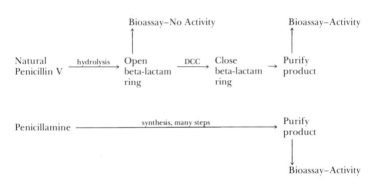

Plan of relay synthesis.

I began with natural penicillin V, which of course was biologically active. Subjecting this penicillin to alkaline hydrolysis opened the beta-lactam ring and destroyed the biological activity of the compound. Henery-Logan worked on the opening, following my instructions.

The problem was that when you opened it up, you had to make sure that it was a hundred percent opened up so when you closed it again, you were not showing biological activity left over from the original [penicillin] V. I did this by purifying the opened up product. This was a new compound. A di-acid was recrystalized several times, found to be analytically pure, shown to have no beta-lactam by infrared spectra and more importantly, by bioassay at Bristol labs. So the opened up product was completely opened up. I then investigated the application of the reagent dicyclohexylcarbodiimide to this cyclization. This cyclization worked [Henery-Logan deposition].

This was a critical step in the proof, for we did not want to repeat the classic blunder of the Portuguese chemist who had failed to test his intermediate for biological activity and mistakenly concluded that the small amount of unopened ring he had carried through his reactions was actually the result of his own efforts to close the opened ring. We then closed the ring with DCC, purified the product, and bioassayed. I was delighted to learn that the final product had the same biological activity as the original penicillin V. The reactions I designed had closed the beta-lactam ring and, as a result, reconstituted the original penicillin.

To carry out the total synthesis of penicillin with high yields, I knew that I would need appropriate blocking groups to protect the delicate beta-lactam function, but by and large the most difficult work had already been done. I had learned how to close the ring.

Two options in planning the synthesis were open to me. The first, the unprotected route, was to close the beta-lactam ring before adding the side chain and then try to protect it in various ways so that the delicate spring mechanism of the strained beta-lactam ring did not fly open as it had done so often in the past. The other course, the protected route, was to reserve the crucial operation of closing the ring for the final stages of the synthesis. I could protect the elements of the beta-lactam with blocking groups and remove the protection just before we were ready to close the ring.

I worked simultaneously on the unprotected route and the protected route. However, the unprotected route was the simpler and more direct approach to the problem. Occam's famous dictum that logical steps should be added to a proof only out of necessity (*entia non sunt multiplicanda praeter necessitatem*) is as applicable to organic chemistry as it was to divine metaphysics. Seek the simplest solution. In other words, in planning the series of steps by which to synthesize penicillin, I felt we should not unnecessarily multiply the chemical operations. Each step of the process could introduce new potential problems; and in a synthesis involving several complicated steps, problems could multiply intolerably.

The success of the protected route depended on my choice of blocking groups. In organic chemistry, a blocking group (sometimes called a protecting or masking group) is used to cover a potentially reactive function on the molecule so that one can carry out an operation on another part of the molecule. When the chemist has sufficiently changed the conditions of the reaction so that the unwanted reaction can no longer present a problem, he can remove the blocking group. By adding and removing blocking groups at critical points in the synthesis, the chemist can direct the reactions as he wishes. The trick is discovering the appropriate blocking groups.

When the synthesis of crystalline 6-APA was started in about March 1959, I suggested using the trityl protective group on the nitrogen and a methyl ester on the carboxyl. Thus one amino group and one carboxyl group would be protected and the other amino group and carboxyl would react. Henery-Logan did it first with the methyl ester on the carboxyl of the thiazolidine ring. At the other end, there was a tritylamino group. The yield in the beta-lactam cyclization using carbodiimides was very gratifying. Work on safely removing the protective groups was complete by the summer of 1959.

Several considerations determined my choice. Compound VIII, in my naming scheme, has two carboxyl groups. To obtain the highest possible yield, the carboxyl group that was to become part of the beta-lactam ring had to be protected until I was ready to close the ring. At the same time, I had to protect the primary amine, lest it react with the carboxyl group to give an oxazolone, as in the Robinson formula. I also wanted to take advantage of the bulk contributed by blocking groups. I knew that the beta-lactam ring was severely strained. To close it, therefore, required considerable work. A force imposed from outside the ring would enhance the probability of the two ends of the ring coming close enough to form a bond. I hoped that a bulky blocking group attached to the primary amine would help push the ring together. Finally, in selecting blocking groups I had to remember that a time would come in the course of the synthesis when I would want to remove the group. Although the blocking group had to bind fast to the molecule as long as I wanted it to, the group also had to be relatively easy to remove when it no longer served my purposes. If the blocking group came off the molecule too readily, I could not count on it being there when I needed it. If it turned out to be too difficult to remove, the harsh treatment needed for removing the blocking group might disturb the rest of the molecule. I was all too aware of the fearsome sensitivity of the penicillin molecule—the bugbear that had haunted all previous chemists in their attempts to close the beta-lactam ring.

I experimented with several blocking groups. The first was the tertiary-butyl (t-butyl) group for covering a carboxyl function, especially during reactions that are neutral or basic. I had begun using it as early as 1950. The t-butyl group is easily added in the form of isobutylene with an acid catalyst. The group is easily removed, too, in a nonprotonating solvent. Even a small amount of hydrogen chloride will remove the blocking group almost immediately.

The second blocking group I worked with was the phthaloyl group, used by Victor Frank in my laboratory in 1949 for peptide syntheses. The phthaloyl group covers both protons of the primary amine and is removed easily at the proper time. The group is very stable under acid and neutral conditions, but it will readily come off the molecule when treated with hydrazine without disturbing the rest of the molecule. This reaction also will take place under mild conditions.

The third blocking group I used was the trityl group (otherwise known as triphenylmethyl). Professor Zervas, at the University of Athens, had developed this group for covering an amine. I attached this trityl group to the amine but got much more mileage out of it than simply to use it as a blocking group. This bulky group—three big six-carbon rings surrounding a carbon atom—would be just the lever I needed to help push the beta-lactam ring closed. Moreover, because the trityl group resists treatment by sodium hydroxide (saponification), it further stabilizes the beta-lactam. Finally, by being attached to the primary amine, the trityl group prevents the formation of the oxazolone. The carboxyl group could not swing around to form a bond with the primary amine; it had to form the beta-lactam. To remove the trityl group was no problem either. Treatment with dilute acetic acid, for instance, would take it off.

Finally I selected three new blocking groups for the synthesis of penicillin. Using these new techniques, I could run the last eight steps of the penicillin synthesis at or below room temperature, which meant that the reactions could proceed under extremely mild conditions. To cover the penicillamine carboxyl group I used either methyl or, better, benzyl. The carboxyl group that formed the beta-lactam ring was protected by t-butyl. I used diisopropylcarbodiimide to close the beta-lactam ring rather than the DCC, which we used earlier in the peptide synthesis and in the early stages of our penicillin work, because it is relatively volatile and on freeze-drying the mixture eliminates the excess reagent. This cyclization gave approximately a 70 percent yield; in fact, in all the synthetic steps in the total synthesis no yield was lower than approximately 70 percent, and some were close to quantitative.

The effect of the bulky trityl group is to enhance the ring closure. It is well known that bulky substituents on a small ring help the ring closure. The next step is something that would have amazed most penicillin chemists: we simply saponified the methyl ester without affecting the beta-lactam ring seriously and this again was made possible by the bulky trityl group. In more recent work, I used the benzyl group and some other ester groups on the carboxyl function and have obtained still higher yields. This produces 6-APA, which we then condense with various acid chlorides and other acylating agents. All this work was reported in London in the spring of 1958; it had all been completed in 1956–1957.

Naturally in the course of such a difficult and complex synthesis, I ran into a fair number of dead ends and other practical frustrations. Often I found myself at an impasse. I knew, however, that the only thing to do at such times is to back up and try another approach. Finally I put together a series of reactions that yielded the prize. Over the years, I refined the methods; but the following are the basic strategies of synthesizing penicillin by wholly chemical means. The outline of the reactions looks simple enough, but in practice the synthesis of penicillin is still a formidable task.

### Success

My discovery met with mixed reactions. The popular press, not always the most accurate reflection of the value of a scientific discovery, announced that I had "devised a practical method of producing the penicillin molecule synthetically" and predicted that "the announcement will have far-reaching effects in the pharmaceutical industry" (*Business Week*, 1957). *Time* more soberly reminded its readers that "there is little chance that Sheehan's method will be used to

Synthesis of penicillin.

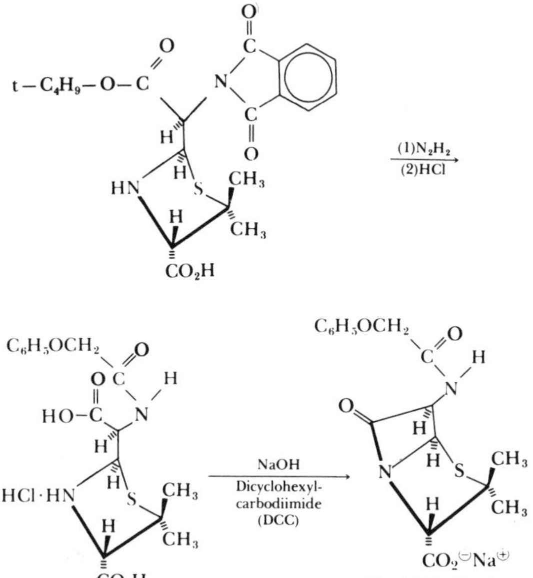


Penicillin V salt

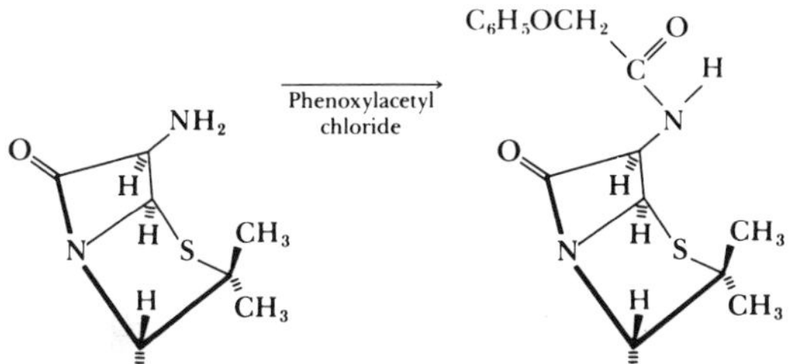


Sodium salt of 6-APA

Penicillin V

manufacture penicillin V commercially, since it can be made cheaply by fermentation." Nevertheless, *Time* said, the discovery was an important one because it allowed the possible production of new artificial penicillins.

I continued to improve upon the reactions. The yield of that first series, going by the unprotected route, was no more than 1 percent. But even that small yield was significant because it showed that penicillin V could be synthesized by a *rational* chemical process. Having synthesized the compound by a chemical process that was planned in advance and, therefore, well understood, meant that I could work on the reactions to improve the yield. By 1959 my laboratory was obtaining yields of 60 to 70 percent.

By the end of 1959, Ernst Chain, the skeptic of only a few years earlier, announced to the world that a new age of penicillin research had dawned. "I think," he is quoted as saying (*New York Times*, October 27, 1959, p. 7), "we've entered a completely new era in this penicillin field, and I think we can look ahead with bright new optimism."

Two factors contributed to Chain's renewed enthusiasm: my own work and work in which Chain was involved. Beecham, a British firm, became interested in the penicillin field at just about the time I was finishing my penicillin synthesis. They discovered how to produce large quantities of 6-APA; I had developed a variety of chemical techniques for acylating it. In the spirit of the new age, Beecham and Bristol agreed to join in a venture producing synthetic and semisynthetic penicillins. Two scientists represented Beecham at those early meetings in April 1959, Doyle and Rolinson. Included among the scientists representing Bristol were Sheehan, Menotti, Cheney, and Lein.

# 6  *Ordinary Skill in the Art*

Patents are granted, according to the Constitution of the United States, "to promote the progress of science and the useful arts by securing for limited times to authors and inventors the exclusive rights to their respective writings and discoveries" (Article 1, section 8). However, the climate of science has changed considerably in the roughly two hundred years since the Founding Fathers wrote those words. Then Thomas Jefferson recognized the value to the commonweal of a steady progress in the sciences and therefore protected the processes of invention. In my own case, rather than the sweetness and light promised by the noble words of the Constitution, patent issues embroiled me in a process at least as difficult and far more contentious than the entire effort to synthesize penicillin.

We have already seen how contending forces seriously hampered the original OSRD penicillin synthesis program. Academic and industrial scientists battled over their relative stature in the scientific community; government officials and commercial managers fought over the organization and administration of the project; and commercial interests and nonprofit institutions haggled over money. Once we had accomplished the long-awaited feat of synthesizing penicillin, the scientific struggle was suspended, and the most pressing issues became the valuable patent rights to what promised to be a vast number of newly developed penicillins. At the beginning of the penicillin era, industrial and scientific interests were poised for battle over the new antibiotic, and the legal mechanisms were not yet sufficiently refined for dealing with the contests.

After the close of the OSRD program, the issue of patents had, to a large extent, been brushed under the rug. Commercial interests involved in the penicillin synthesis program had agreed to waive all patent claims until the cessation of the war and termination of the government project. Bush and Richards were empowered to distribute patent rights among the parties involved. The distribution process was complex, and its chances of working were limited.

Add to this mixture of problems matters of national honor, industrial zeal, and personal pride, for many people in Britain came to hold the opinion that American firms were growing rich on Fleming's original discovery and Florey's development of it. More than once the charge has been made that Florey handed the penicillins over to the Americans. In response to that charge Karl Folkers said, "I know I've heard that many, many times, but I think the later trouble all grew out of the governmental cooperation between Washington and the British group." I agree with Folkers. The tangle of personal and commercial motives, of necessity ignored during the active years of the OSRD penicillin synthesis project, became increasingly important as the value of penicillin inventions became apparent.

The most important penicillin invention of them all, certainly, was the invention of methods for producing the nucleus of the penicillin molecule—free 6-APA. Much of the patent fight I found myself caught up in involved processes for preparing and acylating free 6-APA.

The rules of patent law do not grant patent protection to what already exists and is known. The important tests of the validity of a patent, therefore, are novelty, utility, and invention. "Whoever invents or discovers any new and useful process, machine, manufacture, or composition of matter, or any new and useful improvement thereof, may obtain a patent therefor" (Section 101, 35 USC of the Patent Act of

1952). "The specification shall contain a written description of the invention, and of the manner and process of making and using it, in such full, clear, concise, and exact terms *as to enable any person skilled in the art* [emphasis added] . . . to make and use the same" (Section 112).

Jurists argued during the 1940s that a principle of nature did not come under this legal definition of an invention. When an inventor prepares a chemical compound, according to patent authorities, natural forces are ultimately responsible for the particular chemical structure achieved. More recently, however, patent doctrine has been broadened. Although it cannot be denied that natural forces are ultimately responsible for the combinations of atoms in chemical structures, a particular structure deliberately formed by a chemist in the laboratory is a product of art and not a product of nature. Any "new and useful" chemical product, consequently, may now qualify as an invention.

An early instance of the difficult reasoning involving patents of natural products is the famous case of the patent covering a method for producing vitamin $D_3$. Dr. Harry Steenbock prepared vitamin $D_3$ by irradiating 7-dehydrocholesterol, a precursor of vitamin $D_3$ available as a naturally occurring substance or prepared easily from other steroids. Steenbock received a patent for his procedure and then donated the patent to the Wisconsin Alumni Research Foundation. The original funding of that foundation, in fact, derived in large part from the Steenbock patent.

Unfortunately for the foundation, however, the Steenbock licensing agreement contained a clause that required the holder of the patent to prosecute anyone who might infringe the patent. Usually a holder of a patent will not go after a small infringer unless he becomes a serious competitor because patent proceedings ordinarily take far too much time and money to warrant such vigilance. The Wisconsin group, however, was forced by the terms of the licensing agreement to prosecute a small West Coast firm that was selling vitamin D prepared roughly by the Steenbock irradiation method. As a result, the Wisconsin group lost the patent. The defense of the infringer was that natural 7-dehydrocholesterol was known to occur in sheep wool and that sheep could be readily observed in the pasture under natural sunlight. Those sheep commonly lick their fleece and, therefore, according to the finding of the court, those sheep had anticipated the Steenbock patent.

To qualify as a patentable substance, a naturally occurring compound must require the exercise of art and ingenuity to make that compound available for use. By this line of argument, such apparently natural substances as testosterone produced in the testes, streptomycin produced by soil bacteria, hybrid corns, and the American Beauty rose can all be patented as artificial substances. Thus the chemical equivalent of a natural product such as penicillin, prepared by human ingenuity by a novel chemical process, can be patented also.

When the Oxford group first isolated penicillamine in 1943, Florey and Chain were quick to see the commercial possibilities of their invention. In his London News-Letter (No. 63, October 9, 1943), Joseph W. Ferrebee wrote,

Chain and the Oxford group have established by synthesis the structure of one of the portions of the penicillin molecule. Details of their observations and method of synthesis of penicillamine will be sent to Dr. Richards. Chain is very anxious that this information be treated as a "disclosure" and not as a publication in the patent sense. The question of ultimate patent problems has not been clarified here, and it is hoped that information sent to the States will be handled in a manner which will not compromise the eventual obtaining of patents on some of these processes.

On the basis of this early success, Chain had believed that penicillin would be synthesized within the next few months and was therefore eager to establish his patent position. According to their colleague at Oxford, Edward Abraham, both Florey and Chain were eager for a patent. Chain was especially eager because, as Abraham said, "he came from an industrial chemical background. It was a world with which he was familiar. The problem was that the official attitude toward the taking of patents by academic people in medical, academic research was very much against it. The Medical Research Council made it clear that they would be very much opposed. There was no mechanism whereby they would be willing to help."

Because a patent grants an inventor exclusive right to "make, use, or vend" his invention for seventeen years, there has been considerable ambivalence about the propriety of patenting a medical invention or discovery. This ambivalence is especially poignant in the universities, where dedication to even the purest research in the pursuit of knowledge may nevertheless lead to practical inventions.

One of the factors responsible for the attention university administrators paid to inventions in the field of medicine was the famous case of the Drinker respirator. Professor Phillip Drinker and his brother Cecil, at Harvard, developed a prototype of the mechanical respirator, known as the iron lung. Even with his relatively primitive machine, known to this day as the Drinker respirator, physicians were able to maintain life in cases of respiratory paralysis. Before the advent of polio vaccines to prevent the disease, the Drinker respirator was probably responsible for saving the lives of many polio victims.

After considerable discussion with Harvard, Professor Drinker chose to take out a patent on the machine and independently went into commercial production. At that moment, a vigorous and, in my opinion, unjustified outcry went up from the press and academic community. The popular judgment was that a device such as his, capable of saving lives and developed in a nonprofit academic institution, should not be patented for private gain.

The Drinker precedent was used by many universities to say that any invention in the public health area should not be patented or, if it were, the patent should be dedicated to the public. The result of this restrictive ruling was that, to a large extent, medical invention in the universities was curtailed. At the time of our penicillin work, for example, MIT was strongly inclined to follow the Drinker precedent. In fact, when I first synthesized penicillin, in 1957, MIT was reluctant to protect my invention with a patent. Only after I said that I would take out my own patent did MIT act.

Since I was convinced in early 1957 that a patent should be applied for, I reported the situation to the MIT Patent Committee, of which Professor Carl F. Floe was then chairman. Apparently the Patent Committee recognized that penicillin presented an unusual situation as well as one with considerable potential for arousing public attention, for Professor Floe consequently referred the matter to James R. Killian, who was then president of MIT.

After I had outlined my position in some detail to President Killian, he asked me, "John, do you think that we should take out a patent on this?" I was somewhat startled by his question, but I said that I certainly did think that somebody should take a patent on the synthesis of penicillin. I knew that commercially useful processes would be developed from our work, and that if we did not take out the patent, someone else would. I remember saying to President Killian, "I think the patent should certainly go to the organization that developed the invention."

President Killian gazed for a long moment out the window. I will never know what he was thinking, but his next comments suggested that he was thinking of Drinker. "John," he said, "if this were in any area but public health, I would give you the patent. You could take it out on your own. But since your invention is in the area of public health, I feel that MIT should take out the patent."

## Fight over the Patent

Jeff Wylie, head of public relations for MIT, called me one morning in 1959, soon after news of my improved synthesis had been picked up by the news media. "John, are you sure that you really synthesized penicillin?" he asked. I managed to assure him that I was quite sure. "We have several reports of the synthesis in publication," I said, "and we have years of research data to back up the reports. I can produce samples of our compounds. Why do you ask me such a curious question?" His reply was even more startling than his initial question. "The British Ambassador has been in touch with the U.S. State Department, and the State Department has just called our office. The British want to know if you really did accomplish the synthesis that has been publicized in the newspapers. They feel in the British Embassy that the publicity you are getting takes some of the thunder from their own recent successes in the penicillin field."

Clouded judgment seems to have attended almost every phase of the penicillin development. In the early days, the beta-lactam ring confounded the best chemists of our generation so that many years elapsed before the proper chemical formula could be assigned to the compound. In the later days of penicillin development, too, the tricky chemistry of the beta-lactam made penicillin a formidable problem to work on. Finally, in the commercial exploitation—and all the scientific, legal, and financial activities that must accompany the industrial development of a valuable product—perhaps we see the most notable examples of how normally sober and reasonable people were bewitched by the enchantment of penicillin.

British inquiries went no further, and I did not investigate further what the British authorities might have wanted. To the best of my knowledge, this minor international incident is simply another indication of the immense proprietary interest the British maintained in the development of penicillin.

Amel Menotti called me in early January 1959, suggesting that I not visit Syracuse that month for my regular consulting trip to Bristol. He would only tell me, by way of explanation, that Bristol was in the midst of complex negotiations with another pharmaceutical company on a very interesting development in the penicillin field. Menotti did not name the other company and he would not disclose further information about the interesting development. I guessed, however, that Bristol was probably talking with some group that had developed a commercial method for obtaining free 6-APA. This was quite a surprise to me because I was not aware of any other group—academic or industrial—that was carrying out totally synthetic work in this area.

Amel Menotti's telephone call reminded me of a similar situation some years earlier. Max Tishler, research director of Merck and Company, telephoned me in the early 1950s to say that a Portuguese chemist had claimed to have synthesized penicillin and had sent a 10-gram sample. After careful checking Merck confirmed that the sample was indeed penicillin.

I said to him, "Max, don't get too excited about the 10 grams that he gave you, even if that sample is identical to natural penicillin. The real test of whether what he gave you is a true synthetic product is whether or not it is a mixture of the D and L forms. Ask him to give you even 100 milligrams of D, L-penicillin. If he can do that, you better do business with him."

Of course the Portuguese chemist could not produce a mixture of D and L forms; he had fallen prey to his own careless work. His research plan was to start with a natural penicillin and then to open the ring. Using a strange amine to close the ring, he hoped to show that he could synthesize penicillin chemically. When he ran his final assay for biological activity, he did find about 5 or 10 percent penicillin. In the first heat of success, he reported his results to Merck. However, he had not purified his products adequately, and the small amount of activity in the final product was actually 5 or 10 percent of unopened beta-lactam carried from the original sample through to the end of the synthesis.

Amel Menotti's news was considerably more substantial. He was not merely transmitting news of a possible competitor but stating that Bristol had already begun discussion with a very real competitor. Dr. Menotti suggested that I clarify my patent position so that I would feel free to enter into technical discussions with the new group. I informed Dr. Menotti that I would try to put my own patent work at MIT in order, bringing it up to date with the view of possibly cooperating in penicillin research projects Bristol might carry out with the still unidentified group.

Eventually I was informed that the mystery group was Beecham Laboratories in England. Scientists there found a way to isolate relatively pure 6-APA from the fermentation broth. After considerable investigation, microbiologists outside the Beecham group learned that the 6-APA nucleus is not the actual precursor of penicillin in living systems. Rather, what Beecham managed to do was interrupt the natural process in such a way that 6-APA is a useful by-product of the still mysterious process by which microorganisms acylate an unknown chemical precursor to form penicillin. Beecham also developed methods for removing the side chains from penicillins by the use of enzymes. The result was that Beecham had devised a way to produce massive amounts of relatively inexpensive 6-APA.

Who was Beecham? By the mid-1950s, Beecham had developed a strong line of proprietary products. In the field of patent medicines, they sold Beecham's Powders, Phensic, Macleans' indigestion remedies, and a candy called MacSweets. They also had a line of toilet products that included shampoos and Macleans' Peroxide Tooth Paste. Perhaps their largest selling item was the hair dressing Brylcreem. In 1956, Beecham sold 60 million packages of this product. They also sold a variety of proprietary foods and beverages. In the ten-year period ending in 1956, Beecham's group sales doubled. The company was looking for new fields to cultivate. Thus sometime in the mid-1950s Beecham decided to enter the lucrative field of ethical drugs.

Professor Ernst Chain, who was then working as principal investigator at the Instituto Superiore di Sanita in Rome, was retained by Beecham as a consultant. Beecham apparently also arranged for Chain to train Beecham personnel in the Italian laboratory. Although Chain was trained as an organic chemist, he became much more interested in the fermentation field. This was the work he continued in Italy. One of the new Beecham employees to work with Chain in Italy was George Rolinson, a microbiologist hired to get Beecham into the penicillin field. Rolinson went to Rome to learn Chain's latest techniques for fermentation of *Penicillium*; and after his stint in Chain's laboratory, Rolinson went back to England to work in the newly established research laboratories of Beecham.

Chain's advice to Rolinson and the rest of the Beecham research staff was peculiar. He urged them to investigate a new penicillin that had recently been described by a group of Canadian workers. This penicillin, which could be called para-aminopenicillin G because it differed from penicillin G only in having the additional para-amino group on the aromatic ring, was not at all promising for use as an antibiotic. It is rather strange, therefore, that Chain would recommend their working on such a difficult compound. Nevertheless, Rolinson and others at Beecham Laboratories eagerly began work on this new penicillin. In a short time, they realized that they would have serious difficulties in isolating the new penicillin, and their work slowed.

Before going on with the story, I must digress to give a bit of historical background. One of the chemical tests that had been used to determine the concentration of penicillin in a sample involved the treatment of a penicillin sample with hydroxylamine. This reagent converts the beta-lactam to a hydroxyamic acid very rapidly. The reaction of ferric ion with the hydroxyamic acid produces a bright reddish color. Measuring intensity of this color with a spectrophotometer determines quantitatively the concentration of penicillin in the sample. Although the hydroxylamine test worked well when applied to pure penicillin G, when applied to the mixture of compounds present in the fermentation broth, the results were consistently 10 or 15 percent higher than results obtained from microbiological assays. Everyone in the penicillin industry assumed that the microbiological assays were correct and introduced a calibration factor to make the chemical results conform to the biological findings.

It is a curious commentary on the fallibility of scientific thought that the presence of 6-APA in the fermentation broth should have gone undetected for so long. By hindsight, the failure of both microbiologists and chemists to investigate the discrepancy between the microbiological assays and the hydroxylamine test is in itself a curious phenomenon.

Why was the discrepancy not investigated earlier? The answer is simple. It was assumed that some material in the complex mixture of substances found in the fermentation broth, probably an ester, was elevating the figures obtained by the hydroxylamine test. Since the substance in the broth showed no detectable biological activity, it was therefore considered a potentially interesting research question but not one of immediate importance. Whatever the mysterious substance in the broth, it was not interfering with the laboratory or industrial processes. In short, there was no apparent reason to go after that unknown factor responsible for the discrepancy between the two tests. It was only after the discovery of 6-APA in the broth that we realized that the entire penicillin industry had been dumping 6-APA worth millions of dollars and pounds sterling down the drain.

Hindsight might lead us to marvel that the detection of 6-APA in the broth being dumped took so long in the industrial setting. Discoveries reflect opportunity, and those working daily with fermentation broth had the greatest opportunity.

In my laboratory at MIT, I had shown that free 6-APA could exist. My research had also shown that 6-APA could be acylated to yield a penicillin. The generic term now in common use, penicillanic acid, derived from my naming system (Sheehan et al., 1953).

Beecham scientists published two methods for preparing free 6-APA. One method involved depriving *Penicillium* of essential precursors; the other method involved removing the side chain from penicillins enzymatically. Four other laboratories developed similar procedures. Beecham's innovations have now been superseded by more direct chemical means, but at the time they were a striking development.

Max Tishler's group at the Merck Cherokee plant in Danville, Pennsylvania, was interested in the processes of penicillin fermentation. They wanted to be sure that their present fermentation processes were working satisfactorily. Furthermore they had hoped to improve the rate of fermentation, the yields of penicillin, and so forth. After Beecham published the 6-APA work, one of the Merck microbiologists at the Cherokee plant came to Max with his notebooks.

"You know, I knew this all along," he said. "I knew there was something like 6-APA in the broth." Indeed the notebooks showed that he was getting *higher* yields by reusing the spent liquor of penicillin fermentation than by using fresh fermentation broth. In his notebook he had written "Could it be that some of the necessary precursor is in there?"

Meanwhile, as an aid in isolating the difficult para-aminopenicillin G, it occurred to the Beecham group to add an acylating agent—for example, acetic anhydride, which is capable of acylating an amine in aqueous solution. When they assayed the broth, both before and after the acylation, they were surprised to find that the microbiological assay went up about 10 or 15 percent after acylation.

Someone at Beecham—it is not entirely clear who it was, as four names appear on the patent—suggested that there must be something in the broth that became like a penicillin on acylation but had little or no antibiotic activity itself. Further experimentation led the Beecham group to apply hastily for a patent in August 1958, suggesting that they had found a way of producing 6-APA.

In the meantime, I had begun to establish my own patent position in the penicillin field. Early in February 1959, I had the attorney for the Research Corporation, Mr. Stowell, take the necessary patent action so that I could freely enter into a cooperative arrangement with Bristol and the as yet un-identified mystery group. The continuation-in-part of my earlier application, dated March 1, 1957, revealing 6-APA and its acylation, was filed by Mr. Stowell, of the Washington, D.C., law firm Stowell & Stowell, patent attorneys for the Research Corporation.

The Research Corporation had been organized to manage patents and also to prosecute the patents for a large number of universities, among them MIT. Their first important patents were those for the Cottrell precipitator, an early device for scrubbing atmospheric pollutants and other contaminants out of industrial exhausts. MIT had placed Professor Jay Forrester's invention of memory systems for electronic computers with them; and MIT thought that the Research Corporation would be an appropriate firm to handle the Sheehan patents as well.

I had met Mr. Blake Yates, vice president of the Research Corporation, through a mutual friend. But despite this amicable introduction, my contacts with that firm were not entirely satisfactory. It seemed to me that the Research Corporation was not prosecuting our application with sufficient vigor. Even more important, they were not entering into negotiations with the groups I thought would be the most likely licensees. I had felt that Bristol Laboratories was our most reasonable choice of licensee; they had supported our penicillin work over the years, and they were very active in the penicillin and antibiotic field. I was sure that Bristol would be fully capable of fulfilling their end of any contract we might establish.

To the end of getting the Research Corporation and Bristol Laboratories together, I talked with the man who was then president of Bristol Laboratories, Dr. Philip Bowman. His offices were in Rockefeller Center, just a few blocks away from the offices of the Research Corporation. I had gone trout fishing with Phil Bowman and Amel Menotti, so I felt that I could ask him to speak informally with Blake Yates. I had also done a little missionary work with Mr. Yates to see if I could bring the two men together.

Shortly after I introduced them the meeting quickly degenerated into a shouting match and name calling contest. Apparently Dr. Bowman interpreted something that Mr. Yates said as a slur on the integrity of Bristol and of Dr. Bowman himself. To my great consternation, Dr. Bowman stormed out of Mr. Yates's office in a high dudgeon and refused to have anything more to do with the Research Corporation. I never could bring the two men back together.

MIT also broke its relationship with the Research Corporation at about that time because of the alleged mishandling of Professor Forrester's patent. I am not at all clear on the details, but I believe that the Research Corporation managed to alienate IBM. MIT asked the Research Corporation to return both the Forrester and the Sheehan patents. MIT then asked me who I thought would be a more successful firm for prosecuting and eventually managing the penicillin patent. I suggested Arthur D. Little, with whom I had already developed a cordial consulting relationship. I knew that they had a competent patent management department. This is what we did.

After MIT and the Research Corporation parted company it was obvious to me that in addition to Arthur D. Little we needed an aggressive and competent firm of patent attorneys to protect our interests. The first two patent attorneys with whom I had discussed the penicillin situation, two men who will remain nameless, expressed the definite opinion that to obtain a patent on something as broad as semisynthetic penicillins would be difficult, if not impossible. They also expressed considerable skepticism about whether the patent would ever be worthwhile commercially.

After Beecham had established the existence of 6-APA and went through the work of acylating the penicillin nucleus with different side chains to form several semisynthetic penicillins, they got word to Professor Chain in Rome. This was the first he had heard of the work. He caught the next plane from Rome to England, to be present at the news conferences that followed. The Beecham investigators who had made the critical discovery of free 6-APA wondered at Chain's efforts to associate himself with their work. His only contribution, apparently, had been to send them off on a wild goose chase after the difficult para-aminopenicillin G.

And so, in 1959, not long after Amel Menotti first contacted me, Menotti, Joseph Lein (head of microbiology), Lee Cheney (head of organic research), Irving Hooper (head of biochemical research), and I represented Bristol at a series of meetings with the Beecham group at their laboratories in Brockham Park, forty miles south of London. Representing Beecham were Doyle, Rolinson, and H. G. Lazell, chairman of the board of Beecham. Soon after our visit to Brockham Park, the Beecham group came to the United States for further scientific discussions. We all felt that a favorable collaborative effort was possible: Beecham could supply 6-APA through fermentation; Bristol had the advanced fermentation technology and the necessary industrial capacity; and I had the chemical methods for acylating 6-APA derived, at least in part, from my earlier work with carbodiimides in peptide synthesis. We were highly enthusiastic, confident that in a short time we could produce a virtually endless stream of important new penicillins.

Bristol dedicated a new set of penicillin facilities in Syracuse in October 1959. Ernst Chain and I were the two principal scientific participants in the dedication ceremony. Our research colleague that day was Governor Nelson Rockefeller; for, at one point in the ceremonies, he turned the stopcock on a piece of apparatus and synthesized a new penicillin on the spot. There had been some minor attacks of anxiety at Bristol over the question of Rockefeller's producing a new penicillin. Some of the bench chemists wondered what would be Governor Rockefeller's claim to a patent if the new compound proved to be commercially valuable. The matter was referred to the Bristol patent lawyers, and long before Governor Rockefeller timidly approached the apparatus we had set up for him, we had learned from the patent attorneys that there was no cause for concern. According to them, "Governor Rockefeller has no status as an inventor. He is merely unskilled labor following directions."

Before the year was out, however, the troika that had been put together in such high spirits was dismantled. Apparently at some point, Bristol and Beecham ran into business disagreements that could not be resolved. More than that, the honeymoon period during which Bristol, Beecham, and I planned for a fruitful alliance, turned into a nightmare of recrimination and legal battles that lasted for more than twenty years. The story of that legal fight begins with my efforts to establish my own patent position in the penicillin field.

I was convinced that using a carbodiimide as the coupling agent was precisely what we needed for a complete and rational synthesis of penicillin. In the autumn of 1956, after many encouraging experiments with the carbodiimide reagent, I asked Ken Henery-Logan to attempt closure of the beta-lactam ring using dicyclohexylcarbodiimide (DCC). Following the outline of our previous work, he succeeded on October 11, 1956. I had him run an experiment, using the utmost caution, in which he started with the natural penicillin V, opened the ring, and then closed it again to show that the carbodiimide would indeed yield a penicillin. In a second experiment, using a totally synthetic precursor of D, L-6-APA, we were thus in a position to close the beta-lactam ring and to acylate to form a synthetic penicillin. Having mastered these crucial steps, we could synthesize penicillin. In March 1957 I suggested to Henery-Logan that he acylate the synthetic 6-APA to prepare synthetic penicillin V.

I had made arrangements with Bristol Laboratories to bioassay the samples. Sample KHL-XVII-39-2 was sent to Bristol on March 22, 1957. The hydroxylamine test and the infrared spectra were run at MIT. I had already estimated that the chemical purity of the compound was about 8 percent. I was nevertheless interested in learning whether even this relatively impure compound had antibiotic activity. The bioassay of VXII-39-2 was performed by Alvin Moses, a Bristol employee who ran plate assays. He was instructed to do very careful work and to take as much time as was necessary. Assay of our sample was treated as an especially important project. In a short time, the report came back from Bristol that our compound did show antibiotic activity. We had synthetically produced penicillin V.

On the basis of the work we had done in October and our continuing work on the acylation of synthetic 6-APA, I filed a patent application (U.S. Patent 643,260) on March 1, 1957, disclosing the synthesis of penicillins from synthetic 6-APA and the preparation of synthetic penicillin V by attaching the side chain prior to closure of the beta-lactam ring. I wrote a good portion of the body of the patent, and Mr. Stowell drew up the claims in proper legal language.

The Patent Office typically acts slowly on such applications. The first thing the Patent Office does is throw up all the objections, reasonable or otherwise, that it can come upon. In our case, a passing reference to work by Kato, Sakaguchi, and Hockenhull raised an objection. The two Japanese references suggested that something they called the "penicillin nucleus," which is attached to the cell wall of the living microorganism, might be a precursor of penicillin. Hockenhull picked up this notion in a review of penicillin research and extended what the Japanese investigators had claimed.

It took us years to resolve the issue. The Patent Office was mistaken in raising objections. Their mistake, however, cost us years of bitter and time-consuming litigation. In many ways, the entire patent fight over penicillin was an argument that should not have taken place.

The Patent Office also complained about the breadth of our claims. Our claims for penicillin were indeed broad. We felt justified in claiming broad protection of our patent because the entire field of penicillin technology, after all, was advanced by our disclosures.

On August 2, 1957, the Beecham investigators, Doyle, Nayler, and Rolinson filed a British patent application (24607/57) for the acylation of 6-APA isolated from the fermentation broth of *Penicillium*. The application was as sketchy as the original research, but Doyle, Nayler, and Rolinson realized their good fortune in finding free 6-APA swimming in the fermentation broth. They never stated flatly what they had or what they were claiming. They were obviously unsure themselves but felt that they should put in an application for the sake of obtaining an early filing date in the event of an interference.

By patent practice, if two inventions are filed within six months of each other, and if these two applications make substantially similar claims, then it is the custom to declare what is known as an interference. In that event, the first group to file an application is deemed the senior party and the later one to file is the junior party. The burden of proof is placed on the junior party; consequently the junior party is at the disadvantage. I understand that the senior party wins about ninety percent of the interferences.

In March of 1958, I made the now famous comment at the CIBA Symposium in London, "We have prepared this compound [6-APA] in a totally synthetic route. . . . We have shown that one can acylate it with various acid chlorides and obtain the corresponding penicillin." This was a disclosure to a select group of chemists and related scientists. It carried two very important messages. One was that 6-APA could exist as a free compound; the second was that it could be acylated to form a number of penicillins.

The 6-APA obtained by Beecham was far purer than ours. In July 1958 Beecham filed a more definitive patent (U.S. Patent 2,941,991), which was granted on July 22, 1958. This was approximately a year and a half after our initial filing, and the normal course of interference would not even be considered. In the meantime, I had been refining my own chemical techniques for synthesizing 6-APA and for acylating it to prepare synthetic penicillins. As I described in the previous chapter, we had worked out new methods using DCC to close the beta-lactam ring with or without new blocking groups. One happy result of our research was that we were able to improve the yield of penicillin from the series of reactions. On May 1, 1959, I applied for what is known as a continuation-in-part of my earlier patent application (U.S. Patent 810,301) and, at the same time, abandoned the patent application of March 1, 1957; in legal terms, I transferred the content or part of the content of the earlier patent to the new application. Thus the continuation-in-part explicitly claimed the 6-APA route, which we had outlined in both experimental detail and structural formulas in the 1957 application.

The battle was on. The Beecham group claimed that their patent should be granted and that I was not entitled to the

1957 application. The Patent Office decided to reject our application as well as the Beecham application, holding them both in abeyance, principally on the grounds of breadth, but also maintaining that the two Japanese references and the Hockenhull review anticipated our claims.

The argument against me was, in part, that my process for acylating 6-APA was obvious in light of certain reports published by the Japanese investigator Kato (1953) and a letter to the editor by Hockenhull (1949). According to the patent examiner, my work had already been done by these investigators, so any chemist skilled in the art could have synthesized penicillin on the basis of what those men had written.

This argument was patently false. To be sure that justice would prevail, I needed good lawyers. After an uncomfortable period of searching, the firm of McLean, Bousted, and Sayre was finally recommended to me, and I made an appointment to see them. I took with me to that meeting in New York not only all our scientific papers and reports but all the Patent Office actions to that date and sheaves of newspaper clippings and other publicity the synthesis had received in the popular press. The *New York Times, Time,* and many other journals had covered the penicillin story. "Behind the headlines last week, about actress Elizabeth Taylor's fight for life against staphylococcus pneumonia," William Laurence wrote in the *Times* (March 12, 1961), "there is a dramatic story, known but to a few in the professional circles of biochemists and microbiologists. . . . What saved Miss Taylor's life was a new drug produced by chemical techniques during the past few months, a synthetic form of penicillin specially designed to destroy the resistant staph germs." The *Times* article continued, giving my "pioneer work" credit for opening "the way to the final breakthrough" to a synthetic penicillin. "It was Dr. Sheehan who, working on his own for two years, then with the support of Bristol Laboratories, plowed on and finally managed in 1957 to achieve a synthetic penicillin." Although the *Times* may have been a bit generous in giving me credit for saving Elizabeth Taylor's life, they did accurately report my fundamental work in penicillin chemistry that led to the drug that saved her life.

I talked principally with Mr. McLean. On examining the matter, he said that we had two choices in proceeding with the case. We could go directly to the Court of Customs and Patent Appeals. That court, he told me, was more powerful than the Patent Office and might give us satisfaction, but cases brought before that court could be argued on the record alone. New evidence could not be introduced at any point in the argument. The other route, he said, was to go through the district court. "I think that the district court is clearly the way to go," he said, "and I think that you have an excellent chance of winning. In that court they will take into account the public recognition of your achievement. Recognition will not be the decisive factor in this case, of course, but the popular and scientific credit you have already received for your invention can be one important element. In the Court of Customs and Patent Appeals, we would not even be able to introduce such strong arguments in your favor."

Mr. McLean said that he would arrange my papers as legal exhibits and put the whole story of our penicillin research in its proper context. "The Patent Office," he went on to say, "is notoriously narrow in its approach. Patent examiners go for the literal interpretation of case law. They look for any little excuse to throw out a case. A court, on the other hand, can take a much broader view."

I had to go to court in 1962 to establish the error committed by the patent examiners in crediting Kato and Hockenhull with anticipating my work. Judge Joseph R. Jackson, U.S. District Court, presided. My star witness was Hans Clarke, codirector of the OSRD penicillin program. For the defense was Joseph Schimmel, author of one of the standard books on chemical patents. It was an all-star cast; the case was a complicated one. Judge Jackson took two years to resolve the issues. In 1964, he rendered his decision.

"The issue here to be determined is the extent to which the plaintiff's process 'would have been obvious at the time the invention was made to a person having ordinary skill in the art.' More particularly, the crux of the matter is whether the references cited by the Patent Office contain subject matter which would have led a skilled chemist in March 1957 to have conceived of the process of synthesizing penicillin in the manner which the plaintiff has disclosed."

Judge Jackson found that neither article could have given the trained chemist the necessary information for synthesizing penicillin. The Kato article, he argued, dealt with biochemical processes within mold cells. The Hockenhull article, he wrote, is "a conjecture on the possible precursors of penicillin in its biosynthesis." Judge Jackson therefore found that "the articles do not pretend to be more than observations of the natural processes carried out by mold cells. They are each predicated upon study of mold behaviour [sic]. The essence of plaintiff's invention, however, is that penicillin can be produced independently of the mold environment." The court also found that if I "alone knew of 6-APA's existence at the time of the invention, it does not appear likely to the court that a process including treatment of that substance would have at that time been obvious to a chemist having ordinary skill in the art."

On July 9, 1964, after "meticulously examining the evidence bearing on the chemical significance of these two publications," Judge Jackson ruled "that the Patent Office has erred in interpreting their meaning." "In this case," wrote Judge Jackson, "it is the opinion of the Court that the totality of the evidence carries a thorough conviction that the Patent Office has erred. Accordingly, the Court finds for the plaintiff and against the defendant, and authorizes the Commission of Patents to issue Letters Patent of the United States containing claims 1 through 7 of the plaintiff's application."

No sooner had I won that skirmish with the Patent Office, however, than Beecham came forward with a claim of interference between their patent and mine. On October 21, 1964, the Patent Office began deliberating the problem of our two conflicting patent claims for the synthesis of penicillin. In the interim, the Patent Office suspended the Beecham application for a patent. On December 1, 1964, I was awarded U.S. Patent 3,159,617. On December 22, 1964, the Patent Office rejected the Beecham petition for interference between the two patents.

*That* should have ended the affair. Nevertheless, for the next fifteen years, Beecham lawyers attempted to prove in several courts that I had not in fact synthesized 6-APA and, therefore, could not be entitled to a patent for synthetic penicillin derived from that 6-APA. On November 17, 1965, Beecham brought the case to the commissioner of patents. The application for a review of the interference rule was rejected. Six days later, Doyle filed a civil action in Washington, D.C., requesting a review of the commissioner's action. Two days later, the court rejected Doyle's case, and Beecham was forced to pursue the argument within the Patent Office.

For three years, Beecham worked at the case. Finally on August 27, 1968, the Board of Appeals of the Patent Office gave Beecham a glimmer of hope. They affirmed the examiner's earlier refusal to allow Doyle's claims of interference, but, influenced by affidavits filed by Sir Robert Robinson and others, the Board of Appeals suggested that Beecham might still have a case. The Patent Office advised Beecham that the best argument they could mount at that point in the debate was one based on an attempted replication of my work. "If they could show that [my] disclosure did not teach what it was alleged to teach, they would have shown that Sheehan was not entitled to the benefit of his March 1, 1957, abandoned application."

The affidavit filed much earlier by Sir Robert Robinson on July 13, 1959, was especially influential in Beecham's case. "I fear no contradiction," he testified in his affidavit, "when I say that its [6-APA] existence was never contemplated. The substance would certainly have been regarded as highly unstable. Its isolation and use in industry was a great surprise and could not have been anticipated by any of the early workers in the penicillin field."

Sir Robert continued, "I have studied [the Sheehan patent] and note that the greater part of this patent has been based on the known work of others, primarily of investigators in the Beecham Group in England, and that the only practical utility of the alleged invention arises from the discoveries of these later workers whose results Dr. Sheehan, the patentee, adopts and seeks to exploit. He does this, apparently on the ground that his synthetic, and commercially inaccessible, 6-aminopenicillanic acid (6-APA) had been converted into penicillin-V by phenoxyacetylation." Sir Robert then raised several technical objections to the conduct of my experiments. He concluded that

"The whole point of this relation of older work is that isolation and proper characterization are regarded as essential by the organic chemist to prove formation of a molecular species even when other methods . . . gave strong presumptive evidence. Sheehan's new synthesis of penicillin evokes the admiration of the academic world, but it is devoid of any industrial importance. It would be a monstrous injustice if the rather "sloppy" experiment I have considered above should be held to give a position which could defeat the efforts of other pioneers who have not only found methods for the production of 6-APA in substance but also used it to develop the manufacture of new penicillins that have clearly proved a boon to suffering humanity.

Ten years after Sir Robert's affidavit, Beecham filed a new set of briefs describing their legal position as of 1968.

Doyle et al. submit that their position from the outset has been, not that the Sheehan parent disclosure is inoperative but simply that the disclosure is insufficient under 35 USC 112 to enable one of ordinary skill in the art to follow the disclosure and produce what Sheehan alleges he obtained. . . . Sheehan admitted that the crucial starting material, 6-APA, was not available as of March 1, 1957 and that it could only have been obtained by following the disclosure of his abandoned parent application. . . . The right of Sheehan to be accorded the benefit of his abandoned application, Serial No. 643,260, and the sufficiency of that disclosure to enable one of ordinary skill in the art to produce 6-APA by the "unprotected route" is thus the pivotal issue in this interference. If the disclosure of Sheehan's abandoned application does not teach one of ordinary skill in the art how to produce 6-APA, the process of the interference counts could not have been performed at that date since the requisite starting material was not available.

Beecham was thus intent on demonstrating that my reactions for synthesizing 6-APA would not work. The question of whether my methods of acylation were successful was largely ignored. If my disclosure could not teach the chemist ordinarily skilled in the art how to prepare 6-APA, the question of acylation to produce synthetic penicillin V was academic. Toward this end, Beecham began a series of experiments in the fall of 1968. John Peter Clayton and J. H. C. Nayler were in charge. On July 28, 1970, Beecham presented evidence that their attempted replication during 1968–1969 had failed to produce 6-APA. On February 18, 1971, on the basis of this report and the affidavits filed earlier by Beecham, the Patent Office declared interference between the two patents. To reopen the case, which had gone through the channels of the Patent Office and the Board of Appeals, and the district court, was a startling turn of events. To compound the confusion, we were made the junior party in the case; that is, the Patent Office had decided to ignore our 1957 application. Because the British filing (August 2, 1957) antedated my own U.S. filing (May 1, 1959), Beecham was made the senior party. However, because of the extraordinary nature of the case, the burden of proof remained with the senior party.

## Inter Partes

The contest between Beecham and me was one-sided from the outset. The Beecham party could subpoena all my papers and any witnesses they might desire. I, on the other hand, was prevented from forcing Beecham to disclose any papers or witnesses they might have sequestered in England. Thus Beecham enjoyed the considerable advantage of presenting testimony about their replication work done in Great Britain during 1968–1969, long before the declaration of interference.

One convenience afforded Beecham by this rule seriously affected the normal mechanisms by which disputes such as ours are adjudicated. In most cases of conflicting claims about a scientific disclosure, the matter is opened for arbitration by allowing the contending parties to find a neutral ground on which to run the critical experiments. In the normal *inter partes* test, as they are called, each party chooses an expert and those two experts select a third, who actually performs the experiment. All parties are present. They are given a protocol in advance, so that they can follow the logic of the experiment and be sure that the experiment is designed to illuminate the central issue of the controversy. The opposite of this two-party resolution of the scientific conflict is the *ex parte* test, in which one of the parties designs and executes the critical experiments. In our case, the Patent Office carefully stipulated that experimental evidence would resolve our dispute only if true *inter partes* tests were conducted.

Rather than follow the letter of the Patent Office ruling and conduct true *inter partes* tests, Beecham was allowed to rely on their own in-house work. Beecham had a modern plant in Piscataway, New Jersey, where they could easily have conducted their replication tests. Eventually they did perform certain demonstrations at that plant, but Beecham chose to rely primarily on work done almost ten years earlier *ex parte* in England. Beecham chose to base their demonstration of the supposed inadequacy of my disclosure on chemical work done by their own employees, well out of reach of any subpoena by us. We could therefore see little of what they actually did; we could only learn what they chose very selectively to disclose to us.

We, of course, demanded to see samples of the products that Beecham chemists allegedly prepared by means of our reactions. Our requests were not honored. A striking feature of the lack of candor by Beecham was their total failure to produce any memos or other organizational documents of almost any description. Attempting to replicate our synthesis must have involved not only laboratory bench chemists but also some pilot plant backup, coordination with the microbiology department, the instrumentation laboratory, and probably several other departments of Beecham. Such a large effort would necessarily require a task force leader or coordinator to bring it off. There is also the matter of money. By its sheer magnitude, the replication experiments must have cost at least $1 million. Anyone who is the least bit familiar with industry, and especially with the pharmaceutical industry, will realize that an expenditure running to $1 million on a problem that is at best difficult and whose outcome is not at all sure would require approval at the highest corporate levels, perhaps as high as the board of directors. Once Beecham had taken their decision to replicate my synthesis, word would naturally filter down through the vice president of research, down to the head of organic chemical research, with cross memos to the heads of the other departments concerned. No such memos were produced in spite of our repeated requests.

We wanted to see more than memos. Beecham was claiming that our chemistry was at fault. We therefore wanted to see what products they were preparing by our recipes. Lawyers for Beecham responded to our legal demands by writing that our requests for samples "not only lack any procedural basis either in the Patent Office Interference Rules or the Federal Rules of Civil Procedure, but, additionally, are totally and completely without any legal force and effect under any case or statute known to us. These documents are therefore *prima facie* without any legal effect and compliance with any requests made therein would be unwarranted, and possibly prejudicial to our client's legal rights." I suspect that Beecham's lawyers took a perverse pleasure in further replying that "Purely as a matter of courtesy, however, I personally would like to advise you that no samples of chemical products designated BRL 7782, 7916, 7954, 7820, 7917, and 7955 are presently in existence to the best of my knowledge and investigation."

The concept of lawyer-client privilege was frequently used by the Beecham lawyers. My understanding of lawyer-client privilege is that the immunity is designed to guarantee frank discussions between lawyer and client. The privilege was invoked in some cases long after the event; in other words, the lawyers came into the story and demanded that Beecham's records that had once been open to our view now become closed.

An extreme example of the extent to which the Beecham lawyers went to obscure the issue is the set of so-called *inter partes* tests finally run at the Beecham Research Laboratory in Piscataway, New Jersey. These were carried out in late July and early August 1977. Our counsel had been pressing the Patent Office to enforce their instructions that Beecham carry out true *inter partes* tests. After many delays, we were finally invited to attend some experiments that Beecham had planned to carry out in Piscataway. We understood, in the most general terms, that the experiments were designed to replicate key portions of Ferris's research work under me. Dale N. Sayre felt that we should accept the invitation, although we were under no compulsion to do so. I was accompanied by Sayre and Ajay Bose. Also present, of course, were Albert L. Jacobs, Jr., the counsel for Beecham, a court reporter, and a Beecham chemist introduced as Dr. Charles E. Windus.

The general atmosphere in which the experiments were carried out was bizarre. Sayre asked what the experiments were designed to show, for instance, and was told nothing. He asked what the protocol of the experiment might be, so that we could decide for ourselves what the intent was, and we were told that we would find out in due time. We even asked what schedule the experiments would follow, so that we could arrange for our transportation back and forth from New York, where we were staying, and again no information was forthcoming from the Beecham lawyers.

At the conclusion of the demonstrations by Beecham's group, Sayre stated,

As to the exhibits offered by Doyle, I object to all of them on the same basis we have objected to the whole test procedure, that there has been no protocol furnished in advance, that the instructions to Dr. Windus were piecemeal, no opportunity by us to review beforehand, and the refusal to designate what particular portions of Dr. Ferris's notebook was being followed. And, as to the APA experiments, we think these are even more improper because there was no notice that these tests would be performed, were outside the scope of the tests you requested to do to the Patent Office; again, no protocol was furnished prior to the tests, so that's our objection to the exhibits and we will move to strike all of Dr. Windus's testimony and the test work on that basis.

The procedure went roughly as follows. Jacobs would ask Windus to perform a chemical operation. "Dr. Windus, what I would like you to do would be to take 50 grams of potassium salt of pen-G, dissolve it in 500 milliliters of methanol and 2.5 milliliters of triethylamine. Then I would like you to let the reaction mixture stand for twenty-four hours." Windus would reach unerringly, one might even say mechanically, for an unopened bottle of commercial methanol. With equal facility, he would open a drawer and find a clean, more likely a brand new, graduated cylinder of the appropriate size. He would reach down and almost magically produce an unopened canister of Pfizer sodium penicillin G. He would weigh this out in the balance and with uncanny smoothness perform the required operations. After Windus performed this operation, we all went home for a day. At other points in the procedure, Jacobs would say, "I would like you to cool the reaction mixture in an ice bath and bubble in 130 grams of hydrogen chloride gas. Then I would like you to let the solution stand for four days." This time-consuming procedure continued for two weeks. Sayre asked, apropos of fair *inter partes* tests, whether Windus had performed this experiment before. The answer was no. However, it was clear to me from the motions that Windus had rehearsed his role several times.

We asked what the point of doing the experiment was, for it did not seem to bear any relationship to work done by Henery-Logan or Ferris. As had happened so many times in the course of these experiments, Sayre was given no information. We eventually discovered that the Beecham demonstrations were not a test of Henery-Logan's or Ferris's work. For reasons that will become obvious, the experimental procedures designed by Beecham were based on a subtle combination of work done by Ferris and Carroll. The Beecham laboratory notebook in which the demonstrations were recorded carried two headings, "Ferris" and "Carroll."

In the final experiment, there was to be a measurement by nuclear magnetic resonance (NMR) of the product that was produced. Professor Bose and I realized, at that point, that the purpose of the experiments was to introduce some doubt as to whether one of our key intermediates had epimerized in the process. You will remember that the stereochemistry of penicillin is difficult and that the spatial configuration of the various parts of the molecule have significant impact on the physiological properties of the molecule. If Beecham could show that our product epimerized to an appreciable degree, they could cast doubt on the entire process.

At one of the key steps in the process, the directions drawn from Ferris's experiments call for cooling the reactants in an ice bath. The reaction mixture must be kept at temperatures between 0 and 5 degrees centigrade, swirled in a bucket of ice and water. In the Beecham experiments, however, according to Windus's testimony, "the cooling bath is a pan containing water with small pieces of dry ice being added to maintain the reaction at 20 degrees Centigrade." The temperature of this system was far from the required 0 to 5 degrees; Windus actually maintained the temperature carefully at a constant 20 degrees centigrade.

When Bose and I learned that the high point of this drama would be to take the final product for testing on the nuclear magnetic resonance machine at Rutgers, we suddenly realized the importance of the elevated reaction temperature. Just a few months before the experiments at Piscataway, Carroll and others at Pfizer Laboratories in Great Britain reported that an intermediate, corresponding to the 6-APA with the beta-lactam opened, partially epimerized rather rapidly at 25 degrees centigrade. The demonstration at Piscataway was designed to permit this unwanted epimerization.

Two different nuclear magnetic resonance machines were available at Rutgers. One was new and extremely sensitive; the other was older and much less sensitive. Beecham's chemist, brought over from Britain to perform just this NMR test, tried the newer, more sensitive instrument first. Unfortunately, it apparently was not working well that day; we were forced to rely on the less sensitive instrument. If the Beecham demonstration had produced no more than about 5 percent of the correct isomer—as the heightened temperature might well have done—the less sensitive instrument might not have been able to detect the desired product.

Furthermore, at one point in the procedure there was a chemical separation, so that the correct isomer might have been discarded if only a small amount of it had been produced.

The NMR spectrum was inspected by Bose, who is an expert in NMR and has published scientific papers and a book in this field. He felt that some appreciable amount of the natural isomer, perhaps less than 5 percent, was still produced. The Beecham group, on the other hand, maintained that no appreciable amount of the natural isomer was produced. I suppose that the outcome of that two-week experiment was moot.

Beecham intended to stop the demonstration at that point. They did not intend to treat their product with dicyclohexylcarbodiimide (DCC) and bioassay the material, which would have been the straightforward thing to do. If they had, they probably would have found that an appreciable amount of the proper isomer had been produced, despite their tampering with the temperatures. This is yet another example of the care with which Beecham selected the experiments to show the supposed inadequacy of our disclosure.

When one goes through just how these experiments were planned and rehearsed, one realizes that they were designed by someone who was a real expert in penicillin chemistry. Curiously, Beecham did not have anyone at that time who was considered to be a top flight expert in the area of transformations and isomerizations in the synthetic parts of penicillin. They were, of course, experts in adding side chains to 6-APA and, more recently, had done other sophisticated work with penicillin. Since I knew virtually every chemist who could be playing in that league, speculating on who might have been the mastermind behind the experiments has been a fascinating exercise.

As a result of our growing conviction that Beecham had not been completely candid in reporting results of the earlier Clayton-Nayler replication experiments, we were forced to take a solemn step. In 1979 we filed a petition "to strike the subject application Ser. No. 870,771, assigned to Beecham Group Limited, from the files on the grounds that fraud was practiced on the [Patent] Office in connection with the prosecution of Ser. No. 870,771." Our claim was that affidavits by Nayler and Clayton, submitted by Beecham on behalf of Doyle and other representatives of Beecham's interests and performed at Beecham Research Laboratory in Britain supposedly to replicate selected examples from the Sheehan patent, appeared to be "grossly fraudulent in that they omitted pertinent data and misrepresented material aspects on which the Office relied." Several of the experimental procedures used by Beecham apparently departed from those set forth in the affidavit claiming insufficiency of my patent disclosure. Results were misrepresented. Significant data supporting my contentions and defeating those of Beecham were simply not reported. Finally, the conclusions drawn from the data reported in the affidavits were false when the data were taken all together. I quote from our petition:

In order to initiate the interference, Beecham set out to prove by *ex parte* opinion affidavits first that Sheehan's reaction schemes were not rational syntheses and, failing that, that replication of selected ones of his examples by one skilled in the art gave no indication of the presence of any 6-APA. The first three affidavits filed by Beecham contained no experimental evidence of their contention of inoperability. Rather, these affidavits were based on wide ranging speculations and in one case, that of Robinson, the affidavit contained little else than vituperations, innuendos and self-praise.

The Examiner in charge of the Beecham application was not convinced by these first three affidavits that an interference should be declared, but he did state that they had presented "expert opinion to raise a *prima facie* question of error." With this ruling in hand, Beecham set out to provide the required conclusiveness of error by replicating Sheehan's examples, the results of which were purportedly reported in two *ex parte* affidavits—one by Nayler, one of the applicants, and one by Clayton, an employee of Beecham. These affidavits relied only on bioassay data to convince the Examiner that the earlier Sheehan patent did not teach one of ordinary skill how to make the 6-APA required for acylation. As a direct result of the bioassay data presented in the two affidavits, the interference was declared.

However, according to the petition, it also became clear "from the interference testimony elicited from Beecham's witnesses" that "the Nayler and Clayton affidavits failed to meet the duty of candor and good faith toward the Patent and Trademark Office." Clayton in his affidavit misrepresented the experimental procedures used, and Nayler concurred with these misrepresentations.

For example, despite my reporting that the 6-APA precursor was a "colorless crystalline material," Clayton consistently carried out his own replication work with an impure, sticky, gummy substance. I had recognized how sensitive the chemical intermediates are to a wide variety of reactions. Separating the product from the solvent was therefore a sensitive point in the process. The most effective means of separating sensitive substances was lyophilization, or freeze-drying. The solvent is frozen as the solution is swirled in a flask plunged into a dry ice bath. The frozen solution forms a thin shell on the inside of the flask. Using a vacuum pump and condenser, the solvent is then sublimed, going directly from the solid state to the vapor. When all the solvent is removed, the product has returned to room temperature; but during the critical period, when the product may react with itself or with other compounds in the solution or with the solvent itself, the temperature is kept safely below that required for the reactions to take place.

In his own "replication" of my experiment, Clayton substituted the older stripping process, familiar to him from his work in petroleum chemistry, for the lyophilization. Stripping removes the solvent from a product under reduced pressure but not at reduced temperature. In fact, as the product and solvent are tumbled in a rotating Buchi evaporator, the temperature may actually rise. Solvent comes off gradually; thus the product is in closer and closer contact with impurities, water, and itself as the stripping process approaches an end point. For these reasons, the stripping procedure is almost guaranteed to defeat the Sheehan process.

Clayton was apparently unsure of the distinction between lyophilization and stripping. "Perhaps," in the words of our petition, "it could be said of Clayton, who was not skilled in penicillin chemistry and who was accustomed to techniques used in petroleum chemistry, that his was a case of gross negligence and lack of skill. However, no such excuses are available to Nayler."

Dr. Clayton testified that his work was initiated in 1968 at the direction of Dr. Nayler—head of the Department of Organic Chemistry at Beecham Laboratories and one of the inventors of the application involved in this interference. Nayler had himself filed an opinion affidavit in the Patent Office in an earlier Doyle application urging that the Sheehan disclosure was inoperable. Clayton was thus assigned this difficult task by his superior who was already on record stating that the disclosure would not work. One can only surmise what Clayton's mental attitude may have been when he commenced his work in 1968. Circumstances such as these have led the Courts to rule that evidence of such *ex parte* tests, if admissible at all, is entitled to no, or little weight [legal citations follow]. . . .

Regardless of any dispute between the parties as to the number and extent of positive results obtained, there can be no dispute whatsoever that positive results were concealed from the Patent Office and the negative results stressed in the affidavits of Clayton and Nayler submitted to secure institution of this interference. We find it difficult to reconcile an objective desire to place the facts before the Patent Office with the concealment of positive results and stressing of negative results in affidavits which supposedly represented the factual experimental situation. While perhaps primarily representative of only the less than careful manner in which

Clayton performed his work, we are also troubled by the fact that the [looseleaf] notebook presented as the laboratory notebook of Clayton was established during the examination of Clayton to be subsequently assembled, subsequently numbered, subsequently ordered collection of papers (undated) which may or may not have represented the full and true record of Clayton work. We find it difficult to believe that laboratories of an organization having the stature of Beecham do in fact normally keep records of laboratory work in this manner. Beecham was not content to use a poorly qualified man utilizing poor techniques with poor materials, but built upon this foundation with poor storage of the test samples at elevated temperatures before analytical testing. The diligence of Doyle et al. in seeking out steps and techniques to minimize the chances of success may not be commendable, but it is certainly consistent and substantial. The list of examples is almost as long as the list of what was done by Beecham. Some others which might be mentioned are, for example, the fact that Bellis utilized a different hydroxylamine test with no standards (Bellis, or course, was not available for cross-examination here); the fact that Shaffner was given only incomplete and misleading data on which to base his opinions; and the fact that penicillinase was not utilized to achieve the more unambiguous results the experts agreed would be possible. As shown by the pattern of examples cited above, at best the circumstantial Beecham record establishes a minimal desire for success and a failure to advise the Patent Office of facts indicating success [brief on behalf of Sheehan, July 13, 1978, pp. 31, 70].

In the outcome of all this fighting, the U.S. Board of Patent Interferences, on February 6, 1979, deftly evaded the issue of fraud. "We do not find any clear and convincing evidence of intent to deceive on the part of Doyle et al.," wrote the patent examiners, "nor is it clear that the Doyle et al. claims would not have been allowed had the Clayton affidavit been more complete and more accurate. We acknowledge certain inaccuracies and certain omissions in Clayton's affidavit which amount, in our opinion, to simple negligence. We do not believe, however, that the ultimate decision of the examiner to institute this interference would have been any different had the inaccuracies been corrected and the missing information supplied. We conclude that Sheehan has not proved fraud or inequitable conduct on the part of Doyle et al. by clear and convincing evidence."

Our evidence was clear and convincing on every other point, however. The conclusion of the board was, "Since Sheehan is entitled to the benefit of the filing date of his parent application, which date is earlier than any date accorded Doyle et al., Sheehan must prevail. Priority of invention of the subject matter in issue is awarded to John C. Sheehan, the senior party patentee."

What could have clouded the judgment of Beecham's management and lawyers to continue their legal fight even after they must have realized that the game was up? In 1974, when we were forced by the courts to show all our research materials, Beecham must have recognized the validity of our experiments and known that we would eventually win the battle. Why did they continue?

One answer, I suppose, is sheer momentum. By the time Beecham had invested so much money and time in legal maneuvers, they could not stop. Perhaps, too, they thought they could gain something. There was always the outside chance that they could play the legal game until the seventeen-year period of the patent expired. If the patent were still in interference, licensing rights might revert to Beecham. This turn of events was not impossible, but the situation was unprecedented in the history of the Patent Office.

More likely, I think, is that a combination of factors contributed to Beecham's zeal in prosecuting the patent case, one of which must have been the national and corporate pride that surrounds penicillin. Charges had been leveled against several British scientists and pharmaceutical firms that they had sold penicillin cheaply to the Americans. Beecham might well have embarked on the legal campaign to vindicate British fortunes, but assuming responsibility for British honor was a unilateral choice.

# Epilogue
## Penicillin: A Molecule Ahead of Its Time

More than fifty years have elapsed since Fleming published
his paper on penicillin; the work by Florey, Chain, Abraham,
and Heatley is forty years old; the total synthesis of penicillin
is almost twenty-five. All that monumental work is now history. The once-heated debate over whether the penicillin
molecule is built upon a beta-lactam or some other structure,
the controversy of whether a series of reactions could be
devised to constitute a rational synthesis of penicillin, the
sometimes uneasy cooperation among scientific disciplines,
pharmaceutical companies, and even nations, the initial
wariness of penicillin among the medical community, and
finally the legal battle waged over rights to patent chemical
processes by which the compound might be manufactured—the many problems presented by the novelty and
importance of the new compound—have now been settled.
But penicillin has not slipped into a quiet middle age. Despite fifty years of study, the penicillin molecule continues
to puzzle and fascinate scientists. Today penicillin research
is more active than ever.

The feat of elucidating the structure of penicillin and
eventually designing a rational process by which to synthesize the compound lay in the deceptively simple problem
of understanding how one carbon atom is bound to one nitrogen atom. When those two atoms are properly connected
in the penicillin molecule, the extraordinary beta-lactam
ring fused with the more familiar thiazolidine ring gives
penicillin its antibiotic properties. When the carbon and

nitrogen atoms do not connect to form the four-membered ring, the compound is not penicillin. Thousands of chemists, biochemists, organic chemists, physical chemists, microbiologists, technicians, and government bureaucrats struggled for years to make those atoms hook up with each other. Millions of dollars were spent from public and private treasuries. But despite the money and labor lavished on the problem, the enchanted ring of the beta-lactam could not be mastered.

Penicillin research was not stymied by this failure, however. Driven by the exigencies of wartime research and the demand for antibiotics on the battlefield and in military hospitals, penicillin workers were forced back on the age-old method of science—empirical observation and practical experimentation. The remarkable outcome of this program, sponsored by the government and by private industry was the discovery of highly productive strains of *Penicillium,* mastery of deep fermentation techniques, and the perfection of effective and economical methods of isolating and purifying penicillin from the thousands of gallons of fermentation broth in which the natural penicillins were produced. While these technological marvels were being performed in industrial and government laboratories, the more esoteric work of mastering the chemistry of penicillin was also going on, often in the same laboratories and by the same people.

Until recently, a clear line has divided pure research from applied research. Industrial research, for instance, relied upon the application of known principles and techniques in ingenious ways to accomplish practical ends. Patents were awarded, among other reasons, for the ingenuity that carried the application beyond what anyone with ordinary skill in the art could do. Inventiveness has been defined in many ways, but they all reduce to thinking what nobody else has thought about information that everyone else has. Pure research, on the other hand, is begun without benefit of the tools and techniques of ordinary skill. The first piece of work, therefore, is to define the problem in such a way that it can be attacked and then to work out new approaches to the problem so that it can be solved. The several years of early penicillin research relied on *both* applied and pure research. Only when the penicillin problem forced chemists into the *terra incognita* of beta-lactam chemistry did it become necessary to devise new blocking groups and, especially, to perfect the carbodiimides as coupling agents to close the ring. With this, industry developed a new life-saving and profitable commercial product; chemistry developed a new area of research.

Future historians of twentieth-century science might well use the example of penicillin to describe the rise of science-based technology, for that compound sits where two lines of historical development converge: one is the ancient folk wisdom about fermentation of microorganisms and the other is the ultra-modern investigation of the *how* and even the *why* of molecular structures and their interactions. Future historians may well see the penicillin program as pivotal research because although controlling the fermentation of *Penicillium* mold was a more or less familiar problem to scientists working during the 1940s, understanding the behavior of the penicillin molecule pushed chemists to the limits of their knowledge. "It has been aptly expressed that, from a purely chemical point of view, the elucidation of the structure of penicillin was a problem of relative improbabilities," wrote Robert B. Woodward in *The Chemistry of Penicillin* (p. 449). "May organic chemists have many more like it on which to sharpen the tools of their science!"

Antibiotics were unheard of at the time of Fleming's discovery, except for a few interesting philosophical questions during the late nineteenth century about life opposing life at the microbial level. As far as was known to those of us who were challenged by the new substance, the penicillin molecule was unlike any found in nature.

Because penicillin was a molecule so far beyond the resources of scientists at the time, penicillin could be studied only by a research program involving the widest variety of disciplines: microbiologists to master the techniques of deep fermentation; chemists to discover effective ways of isolating and purifying the substance that threatened to rearrange and degrade under even the mildest conditions; organic chemists and physical chemists to determine the molecular formula and the structure of the molecule; and finally, synthetic organic chemists to devise wholly new reactions by which to prepare the compound if they were to make a penicillin solely from chemicals taken off the shelf.

One result of this cooperative effort, of course, was penicillin. Another was the newly forged relationship of science, universities, industries, and the federal government. Only the federal government could have organized such a massive cooperative war effort involving thirty-nine laboratories and at least a thousand chemists. Only the federal government could have eased the restrictions of antitrust regulations that might have prevented the collaboration of otherwise competitive industries in their efforts to investigate penicillin and, eventually, produce and sell the wonder drug. Merck, Squibb, and Pfizer—the Big Three of the pharmaceutical industry—were the largest and most influential companies in this effort. They were not alone, however. Once the basic research was under way, another twenty or so pharmaceutical and chemical companies entered the field to produce penicillin and the chemicals needed for its production. Without a carefully defined working relationship among all these companies, the penicillin production program simply would not have taken place.

Taking their lead from the federal government, too, the companies agreed to waive proprietary rights to their discoveries, at least for the duration of the war. In an unprecedented act of faith in the ability of the CMR, the Justice Department, and the Patent Office to arbitrate patent claims once the war was concluded, the companies participating in the penicillin program did share their information freely. Of course, there were times when the old competitive spirit could not be suppressed. But by agreement with the OSRD all companies in the program would allow the OSRD to distribute patent rights to discoveries and inventions at the end of the program. Until that time, all information was to be conveyed to the CMR and shared among the other companies. I find it difficult to imagine a similar situation occurring today.

The cooperative arrangements were not easy to make. Richards complained over and over again of the difficulty of bringing the companies together. However the cooperative research and development program was finally arranged, it is a tribute to the strong personalities of the men leading the program. Richards himself was a powerful and persuasive man, Vannevar Bush was a giant, Chester Keefer could play the role of "God" because he was endowed by his colleagues with godlike qualities. The leaders of the penicillin research and production program took on heroic dimensions equal to the magic of the compound they worked with.

Yet another result of the cooperative effort of industrial, academic, and government scientists in the development of penicillin was the healthy blurring of the distinctions between pure and applied science. One of the classic defenses of *pure* science is found in Henry A. Rowland's attack on empirical experimentation in a bitter address to the American Association for the Advancement of Science in 1883. To Rowland, simple utility had little to do with the goals of science. Rowland refused to "call telegraphs, electric lights, and such conveniences by the name of science." He continued, "I do not wish to underrate the value of all these things; the progress of the world depends on them, and he is to be honored who cultivates them successfully. So also the cook who invents a new and palatable dish for the table benefits the world to a certain degree; yet we do not dignify him by the name of a chemist" (*Physical Papers of Henry A. Rowland*, p. 594). With the wartime development of penicillin—as indeed, in the development of radar, inertial guidance systems for rockets, computers, and transistors—the distinction between pure science and practical applications lost much of its significance.

When science was enlisted in the war effort and, more important, when experience proved that scientific research could make effective contributions to the war effort, the nature of scientific inquiry itself changed. The ancient Faustian equation of knowledge and power was realized as never before. Certainly the most notable example is the Manhattan Project and the atom bomb. In more life-enhancing research, penicillin is another good example. In all cases, however, scientists found themselves confronted by new political and ethical questions, questions they were not accustomed to pondering professionally.

The Drinker precedent, as we have already seen, posed the problems of private gain from publicly supported university research. In another case, also at Harvard, the question arose of allowing the university to exploit some of its research facilities and expertise in recombinant DNA to, in effect, go into the business. This wholly new branch of applied genetics is a potentially lucrative field; and the universities, as everyone knows, are faced with the prospects of diminished resources and rising expenses. Individual university scientists, too, find that their incomes as researchers and teachers do not keep pace with their personal expenses. From a purely financial point of view, economic problems of the institutions of learning and of the participating scientists would be alleviated by allowing both universities and individuals a piece of the recombinant DNA action.

Harvard voted against the idea; the business of a university, they argued, is learning and teaching. Profits are anathema, or at least so difficult to manage that universities are best advised to steer clear of such profit-making activities as commercial recombinant DNA laboratories, computer consulting firms, and the like. Derek Bok, president of Harvard University, is quoted as saying, "These opportunities are tempting, especially today when we appear to be poised on the edge of some vast biomedical revolution. Indeed, the prospects seemed all but irresistible to us when we initiated discussions last year to explore the possibility of helping to create a new commercial venture. . . . However, we slowly came to realize that the path to success would be marked by every kind of snare and pitfall" (*Boston Globe,* April 24, 1981).

Most antibiotics in use today were not discovered in academic laboratories. Two important ones, important for being among the first and for having a lasting usefulness, are the penicillins and the cephalosporins. The earliest work on these profoundly important antibiotics was done in universities. Much of the later developmental work on them was also done in university laboratories. The unpopular research on the synthesis of penicillin, once the OSRD penicillin program was terminated, was carried out only in a university. Because profits are not part of academic research decisions, as they must be at the heart of all commercial research decisions, university laboratories can get involved in long-range, high-risk, innovative research. If the universities do not, who will? Hans Clarke captured the spirit of university-based research in his exasperated reply to the Patent Office lawyer appearing before Judge Jackson. "Money," he exclaimed, "you talk of money when we should be talking lives."

But money is an inevitable issue. History has shown that unless the pharmaceutical industry invests vast sums of money—$60, $70, or $80 million on a compound—very little of real interest is developed. History has also shown that if commercial laboratories are not afforded patent protection, they will naturally withhold their money, and the discovery, regardless of how beneficial it might be, will lie fallow. For example, only when the Supreme Court decided that new life forms could be patented did the large number of companies enter the field of recombinant DNA.

There are exceptions to these generalizations. Wilson's syndrome, a degenerative disease of the liver, can be treated effectively with penicillamine, but in the United States there are no more than 100 cases of Wilson's syndrome in a year. Preparing pharmaceutical quality penicillamine is expensive, and, given the small market for the drug, it is a nonrecoverable expense. Nevertheless, Merck made penicillamine available to the public. Later, however, it was found that penicillamine could be used to treat other conditions as well, so Merck reaped an unanticipated bonus.

In other words, there are no easy generalizations to make about the rules and proprieties of research. The universities, government laboratories, commercial laboratories, individual scientists, and the general public all have rights that must be protected. Each case, probably, must be judged on its merits. The question of how to judge remains.

The broad question of whether universities should be engaged in commercial research is probably too complex and too poorly formulated to be answered. Too many other questions lurk within that question like nested Chinese boxes. A more appropriate approach is to reduce the issue to questions of equity: Who contributed what? Who financed what? Who stands to gain what? Who owns what? These are easier to answer than the big questions of *should* and *should not*. Yet answers are not so simple and legalistic that they preclude ethical judgments. If, for instance, the public finances commercial research, the public should stand to gain.

If penicillin were discovered today, we would probably have the same ethical and legal problems, but the scientific problems of studying a pure crystalline compound with a molecular weight of about 350 would not have been nearly so difficult. Today we have a battery of high-resolution mass spectrometers that, coupled with computers to give real-time analyses, would give us all the necessary structural information. High-resolution nuclear magnetic resonance and natural abundance carbon-13 nuclear magnetic resonance, too, would have been decisive in determining the structure. Single-crystal X-ray spectroscopy and computer analyses of the data generated would have given us the structure in a few days, at the most. The conclusion is that a good graduate student would probably work out the structure of penicillin in a day or so. Just a generation ago, that same scientific feat took the best of us years of intensive work.

The clinical development of penicillin today, however, would be more difficult. When Florey and his group decided that they had concentrated enough crude penicillin to allow animal tests in the laboratory and, perhaps, a few clinical trials on patients in the Radcliffe Infirmary, they started injecting crude preparations of penicillin into patients. It is true that preliminary animal studies in Fleming's and Florey's laboratories had shown that penicillin was remarkably nontoxic to animals and human beings, but the move from animals to people was much simpler in those days.

Today the situation is different: If penicillin were discovered tomorrow, the investigators would have to show acute as well as chronic toxicities in at least two different species. The chronic toxicities may take months. In the case of penicillin, acute toxicities would have been meaningless. It is virtually impossible to administer a dose of penicillin large enough to harm the animal host except by indirectly affecting the electrolyte balance or other osmotic factors. Investigators today would then have to apply for Investigational New Drug (IND) status and begin limited field trials. Volunteers would be selected, Institutional Review Boards would pass on the project, Informed Consent would be elicited from each of the experimental subjects, and throughout all the studies, the research protocol would be under careful scrutiny of the Food and Drug Administration.

Fortunately, penicillin is no longer the pharmaceutical innovation it was just a few years ago. It is hard to recall when chemotherapy was held in low esteem, but the situation in the late 1930s was similar to that of cancer chemotherapy today. The consensus then was that only general protoplasmic poisons would be effective in killing pathogenic microbes and, of course, that general protoplasmic poisons would injure the host cells almost as readily as they would kill infecting bacteria. The discovery of the sulfa drugs, which would react selectively with bacteria, was a major innovation in chemotherapy. Penicillin, as farsighted clinicians were able to see at the time, soon outstripped even the sulfa drugs. As a result, penicillin drugs can be developed today without going all the way back to step one.

The situation is unusual today for medical scientists to accept a chemotherapeutic agent essentially in the form nature presents it to them. In those days, however, the idea of modifying penicillin chemically was difficult to accept. When I made my five predictions of how penicillins could be enhanced chemically, they were met with incredulity.

In the late 1950s, the total synthesis in my MIT laboratories of 6-APA and the acylation of it to form a variety of penicillins, together with the development of efficient microbiological and enzymatic methods of producing this key intermediate, led to the dramatic development of the semisynthetic penicillins. Initiated by the discoveries of Edward Abraham and his associates in the 1960s, the cephalosporins have enjoyed a parallel story. As a result, today one of the major efforts of the drug industry is the chemical modification of naturally occurring substances. In no field of pharmaceutical chemistry is this statement more appropriate than in the very active field of beta-lactam antibiotics. Predictions of how the field of beta-lactam chemistry will develop in the near future are not nearly so simple to make as they were back in the 1950s. We have learned much in the past three decades, and beta-lactam research has gone in many promising directions.

Penicillins and related compounds will certainly remain the most important agents for treating infectious diseases. As we learn more about how penicillins work, we will perhaps finally solve the two most pressing problems in current penicillin research—microbial resistance and patient allergy. One promising lead in this direction is the development of highly specific narrow spectrum antibiotics. Such a beta-lactam compound could be used effectively to destroy one population of harmful bacteria without injuring populations of beneficial organisms in the body. When we have understood the genetics and biochemistry of penicillin-resistant bacteria, perhaps we will have solved the riddles of resistance.

Penicillin research has never been more active than it is today. New techniques and new instruments are applied to the endlessly fascinating beta-lactam antibiotics. Every year new discoveries promise even more astounding applications of this family of wonder drugs. And at the heart of all these wonders is the beta-lactam. After forty years of working with compounds containing that difficult and powerful arrangement of elements, I can say that I have been endlessly challenged by its mysteries. Generations of scientists have now worked on penicillins and close relatives of the penicillins. The more we work on those compounds, the more obvious it becomes that we have only begun to realize the powers locked in that enchanted ring.

# Selected Bibliography

Abraham, Edward P., et al. "Further Observations on Penicillin." *Lancet*, August 16, 1941, pp. 177–188.

Baxter, James Phinney, 3rd. *Scientists against Time*. Cambridge, Mass.: MIT Press, 1946.

Bickel, Lennard. *Rise up to Life: A Biography of Howard Walter Florey who Gave Penicillin to the World*. New York: Charles Scribner's Sons, 1972.

Chain, Ernst Boris. "The Chemical Structure of the Penicillins." *Nobel Lectures in Physiology or Medicine*. Amsterdam: Elsevier, 1964.

Chain, Ernst Boris, Howard Florey, et al. "Penicillin as a Chemotherapeutic Agent." *Lancet,* August 24, 1940, pp. 226–228.

Chain, Ernst Boris. "The Early Years of the Penicillin Discovery." *Trends in Pharmacological Sciences* 1(1979):6–11.

Clarke, Hans T., John R. Johnson, and Sir Robert Robinson, eds. *The Chemistry of Penicillin*. Princeton: Princeton University Press, 1949.

Clutterbuck, Percival W., Reginald Lovell, and Harold Raistrick. "CCXXVII. Studies in the Biochemistry of Microorganisms. XXVI. The Formation from Glucose by Members of the *Penicillium chrysogenum* Series of a Pigment, an Alkali-Soluble Protein and Penicillin—the Antibacterial Substance of Fleming." *Biochemistry Journal* 26(1932):1907–1918.

Fleming, Alexander. "On the Antibacterial Action of Cultures of Penicillium, with Special Reference to Their Use in the Isolation of B. influenzae. *British Journal of Experimental Pathology* 10(1929):226–236.

Fleming, Alexander, and Ian H. MacLean. "On the Occurrence of Influenza Bacilli in the Mouths of Normal People." *British Journal of Experimental Pathology* 11(1930):127–134.

Fleming, Alexander. "Some Properties of a Bacterial-Inhibitory Substance Produced by a Mold." *Journal of Bacteriology* 29(1935):215–221.

Fleming, Alexander. "Antiseptics in Wartime Surgery." *British Medical Journal,* November 23, 1940, pp. 715–716.

Florey, Howard W. "Penicillin: A Survey." *British Medical Journal,* August 5, 1944, pp. 168–171.

Florey, Howard W., and N. E. Goldsworthy. "Some Properties of Mucus with Special Reference to Its Antibacterial Functions." *British Journal of Experimental Pathology* 11(1930):348.

Greenberg, Daniel S. *The Politics of Pure Science.* New York: New American Library, 1967.

Gross, Erhard, and Johannes Meinhofer, eds. *The Peptides.* New York: Academic Press, 1979.

Herrell, Wallace E. *Penicillin and Other Antibiotic Agents.* Philadelphia: W. B. Saunders, 1945.

"In Defense of Penicillin." *Time* 61(May 11, 1957):60.

"Jury Decides in Favor of Penicillin." *Drug Trade News* 18 (October 25, 1943):28.

Levaditi, Claude. *La Penicilline et ses Applications Therapeutiques.* Paris: Masson, 1945.

"MIT Finds Practical Process for Synthesizing Penicillin." *Business Week* 11(1957):124.

"Mold for Infections." *Time* 38(September 1941):55.

"News of Science." *New Republic* 109(1943):20–21.

"Penicillin: An Antiseptic of Microbic Origin." *British Medical Journal,* August 30, 1941, p. 311.

"Penicillin Synthesis." *Time* 69(March 1957):84.

Rowland, Henry A. *Physical Papers of Henry A. Rowland.* Baltimore: Johns Hopkins University Press, 1961.

"Synthetic Penicillin." *Newsweek* 28(November 11, 1946):66.

Thom, Charles. *The Penicillia.* Baltimore: Wilkins & Williams, 1930.

In addition, the following materials cited in *The Enchanted Ring* may be found at the National Archives under the classification Office of Scientific Research and Development Record Group 227, Committee on Medical Research: letters among the scientists and administrators active in the early development of penicillin, minutes of the Committee on Medical Research, memoranda, assorted documents of the OSRD, the Director's Special Subjects Correspondence, regular newsletters gathered by Hamilton Southworth, J. H. Burn, and Joseph W. Ferrebee.

# *Index*

Abbott Laboratories, in CMR
  synthesis program, 92
Abraham, Edward P.
  and beta-lactam ring, 113–114
  and cephalosporins, 127, 207
  in early penicillin research, 3, 28,
    33
  on Florey's trip, 52
  oxazolone-thiazolidine structure
    proposed by, 102
  penicillin analysis by, 94, 95, 96,
    98
  and penicillin inactivation, 131
  *also* 53
Acylation, in penicillin synthesis,
  160, 172, 175, 177, 178, 179,
  184. *See also* 6-APA
Adams, Roger, 88, 89, 90
Adkins, Homer, 112–113
Adrian, E. D., 53
Alicino, Joseph F., 97
Allergenicity, reducing, 133–134,
  208
American Chemical Society Award
  in Pure Chemistry, to Sheehan,
  126
American Cyanamid, in CMR
  synthesis program, 92
Alston, Dr. Aaron, 35
Amidase, penicillin inactivation by,
  132, 133
Ampicillin, and Gram-negative
  microorganisms, 131
Analysis. *See* Penicillin, chemical
  analysis of
Anchel, Marjorie, 90
Atomic Energy Commission, 126
Azlactone-thiazolidine structure.
  *See* Oxazolone-thiazolidine
  structure

Azo compounds, 37–39
  Prontosil, *38*

Bachmann, Werner, 8, 91, 92,
  106, 118
Baker, Wilson, 94, 95, 102, 114
Ballard, Steve, 106
Baxter, James Phinney, 49
Bayer Co., 58
Beecham Inc. laboratories
  alleged patent fraud by, 193–196
  and Bristol Laboratories, 169,
    175–176
  and para-aminopenicillin G, 170
  patent claims by, 173, 178, 179–
    180, 183–188, 192–197
  and patent claim tests, 186,
    188–192
  patent motives of, 197
  products of, 169–170
  replication of Sheehan synthesis
    attempted by, 185, 187, 192–
    193, 194–195
  6-APA production by, 126–127,
    160, 169, 172–173, 179
Benson, A. J., 69, 70
Benzylpenicillin. *See* Penicillin,
  types of, penicillin G
Beta-lactam ring (beta-lactam
  structure), 6–7, 198. *See also*
  6-APA
  anti-penicillinase protection for,
    132–133
  and carbodiimides, 142, 153, 156
  Ernst Chain favoring of, 29
  and difficulty of penicillin syn-
    thesis, 6–7, 9, 167
  and hydroxylamine test, 170–
    171
  importance of, 127, 207, 208

in Sheehan's penicillin synthesis, 15, 152–157, 159

Beta-lactam thiazolidine structure, 104. *See also* 6-APA
controversial discovery of, 113–115
demonstration of, 110–113
proposed for penicillin, 103–104
Robinson opposition to, 29, 114, 115

Beth Israel Hospital, research at, 5

Bickel, Lennard, 57, 58, 63

Big Three. *See* Merck & Company; Pfizer Inc.; Squibb, E. R., and Sons

Blocking groups
definition of, 154
in Sheehan's synthesis, 153, 154–157

Board of Patent Interferences, Sheehan-Beecham decision by, 196–197

Bok, Derek, and DNA issue, 204

Bose, Ajay, 145–146, 150, 188, 190, 191, 192

Bowman, Philip, 174

Bristol Laboratories
and Beecham, 169, 175–176
as patent licensee, 173–174
and penicillin for industrial use, 76
in penicillin production, 160
and Sheehan, 128–129, 150, 169, 175–176, 177
and 6-APA, 168, 169

*British Journal of Experimental Pathology*, Florey as editor of, 30

*British Medical Journal*, and Oxford interpretation of penicillin discovery, 19, 25–26

British Medical Research Council, 56, 63, 81, 165

Bunday, Harvey H., 54

Burn, J. H., 66, 97

Bush, Vannevar
and CMR programs, 46, 74, 86, 87–88, 92, 202
and Merck, 83
and OSRD, 45
and patents, 77, 162

and pharmaceutical industry, 49–50
*also* 72, 75, 76

Business. *See* Pharmaceutical industry

Butenandt, Adolf, 125

B vitamins, and penicillin-synthesis rationale, 82

Carbodiimides, 137–145, 146–149. *See also* DCC
and beta-lactam ring, 142, 153, 156
in penicillin synthesis, 149, 153, 156, 158, 159
and peptide bonds, 137–141, 142–143, 144–145

Carbon dioxide, in analysis of penicillin, 101, 102

Carboxylic acid, in penicillin analysis, 101, 102

Carroll, 190, 191

Carter, H. E., 91, 92, 109

Censorship. *See* Security regulation

Censorship Committee, CMR, 56

Cephalosporin C
and beta-lactam ring, 127
and Gram-negative microorganisms, 131

Chain, Ernst
background of, 28
and Beecham, 170, 175
and beta-lactam ring, 114, 115
on commercial possibilities, 164–165
early penicillin research by, 3, 19, 20, 30, 33
on Fleming's contribution, 20
and Florey-Heatley trip, 64
Nobel Prize to, 18, 27–28
oxazolone-thiazolidine structure proposed by, 102
and penicillamine, 97
penicillin analysis by, 94, 95, 96, 98
on penicillin synthesis, 80, 160
reputation of, 27
and Sir Robert Robinson, 29
*also* 113, 176

Chemical analysis. *See* Penicillin, chemical analysis of

Korean War, and penicillin production, 125

*Lancet*
  Florey reports in, 34–35
  Oxford group report in, 20
Laubach, Gerald D., 150
Laughlin, Joseph M., 41
Laurence, William, 81, 180
Lazell, H. G., 175
Lederle, and cooperative research efforts, 71, 72
Legal issues. *See* Patent rights; Sheehan, John C., patent fights of
Lein, Joseph, 160, 175
Lengyel, Istvan, 145
Leonard, Nelson, 125
Levaditi, Claude, 5
Li, C. H., 138
Lilly, Eli, and Co.
  "admission ticket" of, 75
  in CMR synthesis program, 92
Little, Arthur D., as Sheehan/MIT representative, 174
Long, Perrin H., 39, 48, 62
Lovell, Reginald, 19, 26, 94, 98

McKeen, John E., 125
McLean, Bousted and Sayre (law firm), 180
MacPhillamy, H. B., 90
Mader, W. J., 86
Magee, General James G., 54, 55
Major, Randolph, 11, 12, 70, 83, 89, 112, 117
Manhattan Project, compared with penicillin synthesis, 1, 203
Massachusetts General Hospital, and Cocoanut Grove experiment, 41, 42
Massachusetts Institute of Technology (MIT)
  patent-rights view of, 166
  and Research Corporation, 173–174
  Sheehan at, 9, 14–15, 135, 145–146, 150–151, 166, 167
  and Sheehan patent claims, 166, 173. *See also* Sheehan, John C., patent applications of

Sheehan's penicillin tested by, 177
Matthiesen, C. H., Jr., 88
Mayo Clinic, research at, 5
Medical Research Council, Great Britain, 56, 63, 81, 165
Meinhofer, Johannes, 141
Mellanby, Sir Edward, 57, 63
Melville, Donald B., 117
Menotti, Amel, 128, 150, 160, 168, 169, 174, 175
Merck, George, 75
Merck & Company
  "admission ticket" of, 75
  and Anglo-U.S. cooperation, 53
  biological production by, 70
  and B vitamins, 82
  in "closed corporation," 73
  in CMR synthesis program, 88, 89–90, 91, 92
  and Cocoanut Grove disaster, 42
  and cooperative research efforts, 71, 88
  diligence of, 54
  early penicillin involvement by, 69
  and Florey, 53
  and oxazolone-thiazolidine structure, 102, 103
  and penicillamine, 205
  and penicillin analysis, 95, 111
  penicillin purification work by, 86
  penicillin synthesis by, 115, 118, 126
  penicillin synthesis incentives of, 81–82
  pre-eminence of, 75, 82–83, 88, 201
  research facilities of, 50–51
  research group at, 11
  and Lewis Sarrett, 12
  and Sheehan after leaving, 135
  Sheehan helped by, 129
  Sheehan's work at, 8
  and 6-APA production, 172
  and du Vigneaud, 117
Methicillin, and penicillinase resistance, 132
Meyer, Karl, 35, 87, 96
Microbial Therapeutics conference, 69–71 *See also* Committee on Medical Research

Penillic acid
and argument for beta-lactam,
114
in penicillin analysis, 101, 102
structure of, 101
Penilloaldehyde
in penicillin analysis, 102
structure of, 101
Pennsylvania State College, research at, 5
Peoria, Illinois. *See* Northern Regional Research Laboratory,
U.S. Department of Agriculture
Pepper, Senator Claude, 65
Peptide bonds
and carbodiimides, 137–141,
142–143, 144–145
formation diagram for, 135
and penicillin, 135, 136, 141–142
Sheehan's synthesis of, 135–141,
143–145
Pfizer Inc.
"admission ticket" of, 75
in CMR synthesis program, 91,
92
in cooperative efforts, 71, 72, 88
early penicillin involvement by, 69
importance of, 201
incentives for penicillin synthesis,
81–82
penicillin sales of, 125
Pharmaceutical industry
and CMR programs, 4, 69–75,
88, 89–92, 201–202
and CMR task, 49–50
competition in, 73, 202
and cooperative efforts, 71–75,
88, 201
and government researchers,
73–75
interest in penicillin lags, 76, 123,
125–126
interest in penicillin revives, 127
necessary role of, 204–205
and patent rights, 49–50, 72–73,
75–77, 204
penicillin synthesis incentives of,
81–82
and postwar synthesis efforts,
123, 124–125

Phenylacetic acid
in penicillin analysis, 102
in penicillin production, 68, 69
*Physical Papers of Henry A. Rowland,*
202–203
Podbielniak extractor, 85–86
Prontosil, discovered as antibiotic,
37, 38–39
Protected route, in Sheehan's
penicillin synthesis, 153, 154,
158–159
Protective groups. *See* Blocking
groups

Raistrick, Harold, 19, 26, 30, 35,
94, 98
Raney nickel
in biotin analysis, 118
in penicillin analysis, 110, 111
Rational synthesis
as method, 108, 118
of penicillin, 126, 160, 198
and Sheehan-Beecham patent
dispute, 193
Ratner, 99, 100
RDX (cyclonite), Sheehan work
on, 8
Reid, Roger D., 5, 35
Research. *See* Penicillin, research
on; Scientific research
Research Corporation, as
Sheehan/MIT representative,
173–174
Research safeguards
and Oxford group experiments,
32
and penicillin development, 206
Rhone-Poulenc, Inc., 59
Rich, Daniel H., 141
Richards, A. N.
and censorship, 56, 57
as CMR chairman, 45
and CMR program, 48, 69, 70,
71, 91, 164
and Florey, 53
and governmental researchers,
74
and industry incentive, 49
with Merck, 83
and patent rights, 162

Richards, A. N. (cont.)
  and pharmaceutical industry, 72,
    75, 88, 202
  *also* 46, 77, 87, 89, 98
Robinson, Sir Robert, 69
  on American penicillin contribu-
    tion, viii
  and Beecham patent claims,
    183–184
  beta-lactam structure opposed
    by, 29, 114, 115
  oxazolone-thiazolidine structure
    proposed by, 102–103, 108
  and penicillin analysis, 94, 98
  penicillin synthesis by, 118
  personality of, 104–105
Roche Laboratories, in CMR synthesis program, 92
Rockefeller, Nelson, in dedication
  ceremony, 176
Rockefeller Foundations, 43, 63,
  64, 65
Rolinson, George, 160, 170, 175,
  178
Roosevelt, Franklin D., and
  OSRD, 44, 45
Rossini, Frederick, 107
Rowland, Henry A., 202–203

St. Mary's Hospital, London, En-
  gland, Fleming's work at, 18, 22
Sakaguchi, 178
Sarrett, Lewis, 12
Sayre, Dale N., 188, 189, 190
Schering Corp., 58
Schimmel, Joseph, 181
Scientific research
  pure vs. applied, 199–200, 202–
    203
  questions in, 203–205
  rational synthesis as method of,
    108, 118
  World War II support for, 4,
    44–45, 64–65. *See also* Com-
    mittee on Medical Research
Security regulation
  Anglo-American confusion on,
    55–56
  CMR measures for, 44, 54–57
  vs. free exchange of knowledge,
    55

Semisynthetic penicillin
  Beecham-Bristol venture in, 160
  and patents, 76
  and Sheehan research, 127,
    151–152, 207
Sheehan, John C.
  American Chemical Society
    award to, 126
  and Beecham, 173, 179–180,
    183–192
  and Bristol Laboratories, 128–
    128, 150, 169, 175–176, 177,
    180
  carbodiimide research by, 146–
    149
  career turning points, 9, 10–12,
    14–15, 128–129
  and Cocoanut Grove disaster, 42
  and MIT, 14–15, 135, 145–146,
    150–151, 166, 167, 173
  and moment of discovery, 2
  patent applications of, 166, 169,
    173–175, 176, 177–180
  patent fights of, xii–xiii, 162,
    180–188, 192–197
  and patent tests vs. Beecham,
    186, 188–192
  penicillin predictions of, 129–
    134, 207
  penicillin purification work by,
    86
  penicillin research orientations
    of, 15–17
  penicillin synthesis by, 7, 126,
    149–160, 172, 176–177, 179
  peptide bonds synthesized by,
    135–141, 143–145
  personal characteristics of, 145–
    146, 150–151
  pneumonia-mastoiditis attack of, 8
  and Robert Robinson, 108
  and semisynthetic penicillin, 127,
    151–152, 207
  6-APA synthesis by, 126, 154,
    157, 159, 179
  streptomycin purification by,
    12–14
Shell group, beta-lactam study by,
  106, 111
Simmons, James Stevens, 45
Singh, Jasbir, 141

222  *Index*